Women's Narratives of Health Disruption and Illness

Lexington Studies in Health Communication

Series Editors: Leandra H. Hernández and Kari Nixon

National and international governments have recognized the importance of widespread, timely, and effective health communication, as research shows that accurate, patient-centered, and culturally competent health communication can improve patient and community health care outcomes. This interdisciplinary series examines the role of health communication in society and is receptive to manuscripts and edited volumes that use a variety of theoretical, methodological, interdisciplinary, and intersectional approaches. We invite contributions on a variety of health communication topics including but not limited to health communication in a digital age; race, gender, ethnicity, class, physical abilities, and health communication; critical approaches to health communication; feminisms and health communication; LGBTQIA health; interpersonal health communication perspectives; rhetorical approaches to health communication; organizational approaches to health communication; health campaigns, media effects, and health communication; multicultural approaches to health communication; and international health communication. This series is open to contributions from scholars representing communication, women's and gender studies, public health, health education, discursive analyses of medical rhetoric, and other disciplines whose work interrogates and explores these topics. Successful proposals will be accessible to an interdisciplinary audience, advance our understanding of contemporary approaches to health communication, and enrich our conversations about the importance of health communication in today's health landscape.

Recent Titles in This Series

Women's Narratives of Health Disruption and Illness: Within and Across Their Life Stories, by Peter M. Kellet and Jennifer M. Hawkins

Challenging Reproductive Control and Gendered Violence in the Americas: Intersectionality, Power, and Struggles for Rights, by Leandra Hinojosa Hernández and Sarah De Los Santos Upton

Politics, Propaganda, and Public Health: A Case Study in Health Communication and Public Trust, by Laura Crosswell and Lance Porter

Communication and Feminist Perspectives on Ovarian Cancer, by Dinah Tetteh

Women's Narratives of Health Disruption and Illness

Within and Across Their Life Stories

Edited by
Peter M. Kellett
and Jennifer M. Hawkins

LEXINGTON BOOKS
Lanham • Boulder • New York • London

Published by Lexington Books
An imprint of The Rowman & Littlefield Publishing Group, Inc.
4501 Forbes Boulevard, Suite 200, Lanham, Maryland 20706
www.rowman.com

6 Tinworth Street, London SE11 5AL, United Kingdom

Copyright © 2019 by The Rowman & Littlefield Publishing Group, Inc.

All rights reserved. No part of this book may be reproduced in any form or by any electronic or mechanical means, including information storage and retrieval systems, without written permission from the publisher, except by a reviewer who may quote passages in a review.

British Library Cataloguing in Publication Information Available

Library of Congress Cataloging-in-Publication Data

Names: Hawkins, Jennifer M., editor. | Kellett, Peter M., editor.
Title: Women's narratives of health disruption and illness : within and across their life stories / edited by Jennifer M. Hawkins and Peter M. Kellett.
Description: Lanham : Lexington Books, [2019] | Series: Lexington studies in health communication | Includes bibliographical references and index.
Identifiers: LCCN 2019015804 (print) | LCCN 2019017723 (ebook) | ISBN 9781498592642 (Electronic) | ISBN 9781498592635 (cloth)
Subjects: LCSH: Communication in medicine. | Women--Health and hygiene. | Women--Diseases--Social aspects.
Classification: LCC R118 (ebook) | LCC R118 .W67 2019 (print) | DDC 613/.04244--dc23
LC record available at https://lccn.loc.gov/2019015804

Contents

Acknowledgments	vii
Introduction	1

Part I: Beginnings

1 This Wasn't How the Story Was Supposed to Go: Navigating Unmet Expectations During High-Risk Pregnancies and Premature Birth   9
Jennifer Hall

2 Giving Birth in a Distant Land: Patienthood and Self-Transformation of Another Kind   25
Krista Calvin and Avinash Thombre

3 A Decade Navigating Food Allergies: A Mother's Narrative   43
Courtney Waite Miller

4 Growing Up with a Chronic Illness: Easily Concealed, Even Easier to Forget   61
Kasey Bruss and Jennifer Morey Hawkins

5 Smoking: A Lifelong Legacy   75
Ruthann Fox-Hines

Part II: Middles

6 Through the Glass Darkly: How We Fill a Diagnosis with Meaning   93
Laura Hope-Gill

7 Living with Interstitial Cystitis: An Autoethnography of Developing and Coping with a Chronic Condition   109
Jessica M. W. Kratzer

8	Narrating Menopause with English as a Second Language *Wei Sun*	121
9	"I like to Read, Play Cribbage, Oh, and I have Alzheimer's": Managing Interpersonal Relationships and Early Onset Alzheimer's *Jamie Cobb*	139

Part III: Endings and Legacies

10	Sylvia's Story/The Story of Sylvia: Narrating the Personal and Relational in Patienthood *Leda Cooks*	153
11	Linked Lives: A Narrative Exploration of Positivity and Dialectic in a Patient's Experience *Deleasa Randall-Griffiths*	173
12	A Narrative Account of Father-Daughter Conversations Near the End of His Life *Deanna F. Womack*	189
13	A Narrative Legacy of Family Caregiving *Elizabeth A. Spencer*	201

Index	215
About the Contributors	225

Acknowledgments

I would like to acknowledge all the women who have opened their lives up to the narrative inquiry upon which this book relies. Their willingness to share the deepest and often most personal experiences from within and across their lives, enriches our understanding in many valuable ways. I would particularly like to thank my mother, Mary. In recent years she has given me small glimpses into some of the health experiences of her life that relate directly to me. I was a late pregnancy surprise—the second of identical twins (she did not know she was having twins until close to term). I was her most difficult birth of all four sons (breached). And other such gems! There is so much I have never heard, and never taken the time to ask her about. Working with the stories of this book has inspired me to begin to invite and listen to more of her health experiences and their place in her life story.

—Pete

I would like to echo Pete's sentiments in thanking the authors. Each story in this collection brings us closer to understanding the joy and pain associated with the illness or health condition presented. Many stories elicit empathy while at the same time educate the reader on health experiences, bringing us into the stories as a silent observer. I want to thank storytellers and story listeners of my past and present. From professors who formally trained me; the late poet Dr. James Liddy and Professor Emerita Dr. Pat Stevens—to my folks James and Kathy Morey, dearest lifelong friend Amy Colonna Remillard, and loving life partner Dr. Cory Hawkins. Last, but not least, I would like to thank Pete for guiding me through the process of such a project. You are a wonderful, kind-hearted guide.

—Jennifer

Introduction

This is not an "ages and stages" approach to women's health experience and communication. Neither is it a comprehensive account of the many, or even necessarily the most common, health disruptions and illnesses that women live through. To help organize the book, we draw on the parallel structural archetype of both narratives, and lives, of "Beginnings" (story introduction/ birth and early life, and the beginning of lifelong habits, patterns, or legacies); "Middles" (the body of the story/mid-life); and "Endings," (story conclusion/ageing and end of life communication). This book is organized this way simply to help invite the reader into the narratives—and narration—of women as they live through heath disruptions and illnesses, and story those experiences within the broader context of their unfolding and ongoing life stories. We use this organizing device to help us place communicative experiences of certain types (for example, communication around pregnancy, communication of issues at menopause, or the end of life of a parent) together, and into the broader span of women's lives. We are not trying to pinpoint what women tend to experience at specific stages or phases of a typical lifespan. Rather, we wanted to create a book that draws upon lifespan approaches to communication—particularly in terms of the developmental/ learning and long-term emphasis of this approach (Nussbaum, 2007; 2014)— and which evokes health experiences both within and across bigger spans of experiential time in women's lives, *as they live them*, and *on their own descriptive terms*.

In creating this book, we also willingly traded any notion of capturing the full encyclopedic breadth of possible health experiences that women face, for the rich depth that these chapters pull us into and bring to life for us. It was more important for us to give voice to the various ways that women live through health issues, and the various ways that experiences are integrated into and affect/are affected by their lives and life stories more broadly, than it was for us to document the wide variety of issues women face at any specific points in their lives. In examining women's health disruptions and illnesses within and across their life stories through narrative methods, as we do, we wanted to explore questions such as the following: In narrating health disruptions and illnesses, what communication and relational dynamics, and relationships, are important to women? How do women draw on their experiential and relational histories (and possible futures) in narratively crafting ways through and beyond health disruptions and illnesses? How do women recraft and develop their life stories to integrate serious health disruptions and illnesses into those life stories? How do women's broader, and ongoing, life stories provide ways to make sense of and engage with specific moments of health difficulty? We explicate these questions and concerns as we briefly preview the sections and chapters they contain below. First, we ground this volume in narrative and health communication scholarship.

From before we are born and even after we die, and through everything in between, we are "enmeshed in narrative" (Castellanos, 2013, p. 1066). Writing narratives and reading others' narratives each take time—time that paves a path—a journey through and in time (Charon, 2006). Narratives provide a deeper understanding of how interactions and relationships occur within the context of health disruptions and healthcare settings (Kellett, 2019; Sharf, 2017). Therefore, at the interpersonal level personal narratives are often political due to including impressions of an individual's experience within the broader understanding of healthcare (Harter, Japp, & Beck, 2005).

Narrative inquiry gives precedence to the participant's view, attempting to understand a particular illness or healthcare experience (Patton, 2002) versus favoring biomedical explanations (Castellanos, 2013; Harter & Bochner, 2009). Vanderford, Jenks, and Sharf explain the patient-centered focus of narrative as "a compliment to empirical studies" that allows insights into "patients' sense-making" (1997, p. 23). The meaning-making process of storytelling unearths information about the past, providing insight into how individuals make sense of and attribute meaning to occurrences (Riessman, 2003; Ochs, 2011) essentially bringing the individual to interpret self, relationships, and one's life (Koenig Kellas, 2010). When people tell stories of disturbances to life plans, they include how the instances are understood and reacted to (Harter, 2013). This type of representation allows the teller to (re)frame the "cause and effect" providing the individual the ability to "live in the pain" (p. 9). Storytellers "focus attention on experience and interpret it, creating a representation from raw experience" (Harter, 2013, p. 14) revealing vulnerabilities and struggles.

Storytelling in the context of health situations is a natural and powerful way of sharing "suffering, loss, and healing" (Sharf, Harter, Yamasaki, &

Haidet, 2011, p. 47). Ellis tells us that the act of writing particularly difficult stories is a "gift to self" defining the process as a "reflexive attempt to construct meaning in our lives" allowing us to "heal or grow from our pain" (2007, p. 26). Sharf and Vanderford (2003) add that through voicing the story an individual increases their agency as well as opportunity for healing. The ongoing work of shaping ones health narrative helps individuals make sense of medical situations, and empowers them to own their narrative (Harter, Japp, & Beck, 2005). We have each experienced such empowerment through writing our own health narratives (see Hawkins, 2015; see Kellet, 2017).

Because no two stories are the same, personal narratives of suffering are viewed as original no matter how many individuals might have suffered from a similar ailment, or injury (Frank, 2005). Telling one's story benefits the teller and the reader and/or listener and can be quite transformative for both the "self and society" (Harter, 2013, p. 16). Relational in nature, storytelling calls the listeners to attend to the teller's feelings, often inciting empathic response (Riessman, 2001), ideally allowing the listener to move "beyond our own bodies and experiences to appreciate others' realities" (Harter, 2013, p. 60). Individual motivation to tell a story often goes beyond working out one's own new health status but includes wanting to provide guidance to individuals who also might have a similar experience (Frank, 1995). Powerful health narratives "prove helpful in strengthening the teller's capacity for dealing with illness-related problems" and "awaken listeners or readers to issues that they may not have been aware of or that they are attempting to deal with in their own lives" (Sharf & Vanderford, 2003, p. 23).

Chapters in this book provide in-depth insight into less spoken about health issues. Each woman's story includes how health disruptions impact lives far beyond diagnosis, flare-ups, and/or the individual. Women share detailed descriptions of health conditions that derail usual day-to-day living, adjustments made, and new concerns that arise. Many stories include caretakers involved in the narrator's health story. Several chapters present health narratives from the caregiver's viewpoint, who "create their own explanations of events and experiences" (Sharf & Vanderford, 2003, p. 17). Diagnosis and health issues, whether chronic since birth or newly obtained throughout one's lifetime, impact individuals both in the present and into the future. We believe these stories explicitly or implicitly provide "why the narrative is worth telling" (Bal, 1985, p. 656).

Part 1 (Beginnings) explores spans of experiential time and health experiences that begin in early/younger life. For some women this invokes pregnancy and birth-related disruptions and illnesses, for others it is mothering related, or reflecting on illnesses or habits and patterns that began in their early lives and that will have, or have had, long-term implications for them. In chapter 1 (This Wasn't How the Story was Supposed to Go: Navigating

Unmet Expectations During High-Risk Pregnancies) Jennifer Hall explores women's experiences in difficult pregnancies as they are often quite different from culturally mediated or relationally shared narrative scripts of pregnancy and birth. Hyper-positive and unproblematic cultural portrayals of pregnancy often leave women with difficult gaps as their lived reality can be markedly different from the mythology they consume in popular culture. Calvin and Thombre in chapter 2 (Giving Birth in a Distant Land: Patienthood and Self-Transformation of Another Kind) transport us to Argentina, where Calvin, a young woman who speaks no Spanish and has no family in Argentina must suddenly and prematurely give birth. How does she manage? What helps her and her tiny daughter survive and flourish in a place without her family and support system? How does she turn it into a positive transformational experience despite the challenges? These key questions are addressed as she faces and embraces the experience. Courtney Waite Miller in chapter 3 (A Decade Navigating Food Allergies: A Mother's Narrative) shows us her struggle through complex and mixed emotions, including guilt, and her journey into advocacy for her son who has severe allergies. She navigates family pressures, a medical world that does not always help, and schools that are not always understanding or accommodating. She becomes a wise advocate for him because she had to. In chapter 4, Kasey Bruss and Jennifer Morey Hawkins (Growing Up with a Chronic Illness: Easy to Conceal, Even Easier to Forget) invite us into the reflection of Bruss at somewhere around quarter life, a college student balancing her medical condition and her desires to enjoy the celebratory aspects of college life. She also imagines her life forward. How will her condition impact her long-term desires and life goals as a woman? Finally, in chapter 5 (Smoking: A Lifelong Legacy), Fox-Hines invites us into the daily struggles and adaptations to the breathing related diseases (asthma and emphysema) she now lives with that were caused by smoking, which she began doing at age thirteen (mirroring her mother). With humor and a lack of self-pity, victimage, or regret, she adapts to the constraining oxygen technology and her shrinking world as disability creeps in. She builds a support system that meets her needs and that carefully considers the needs and boundaries of those support system members. Taken together, these chapters show women adapting to reality, navigating complexity and mixed messages, balancing needs and desires, strongly advocating for either themselves, their children, or both, and recrafting their lives around chronic illness that results from health choices made much earlier in life.

In part 2 (Middles) we find women narrating illnesses through memory back into early childhood, forward through imagination into later life, and around them in the present from typical mid points of their lives. In this section we are invited into accounts that show us what communicative experiences and messages these women find challenging, difficult, helpful, and most meaningful. In chapter 6 (Through the Glass Darkly: How We Fill a

Diagnosis with Meaning) Laura Hope-Gill shares with us a poetic account of her journey into deafness. Central to the tale are family memories of place (including sounds), and relationships to the women of her family (grandmother, mother, and her daughter as a mother herself), which mark the phases and changes in her hearing—and the meaning of those changes. In chapter 7 (Living with Interstitial Cystitis: An Autoethnography of Developing and Coping with a Chronic Condition) Jessica M. W. Kratzer invites us into her life showing us how communication enables her to cope with a chronic but not life-threatening condition. Understanding and gaining control of her body, and her treatment, and the freedom and growth this leads to, are central themes. Her story also illustrates how the meaning of IC is one deeply grounded in personal and professional identity and family impact. Wei Sun's chapter 8 (Narrating Menopause with English as a Second Language) focuses on the fascinating current cultural/communicative challenges for women whose first language is not English, and culture of origin is not the United States. She finds such women encountering gaps in understanding and support and being resourceful in stretching and struggling to meet all the personal, familial, and professional demands of life while inhabiting a challenging cultural space. Finally, Cobb and McIntyre in chapter 9 (I like to Read, Play Cribbage, Oh, and I Have Alzheimer's: Managing Interpersonal Relationships and Early Onset Alzheimer's) describe early onset Alzheimer's—a condition that bridges the middle of life to its ending. They evoke the communicative challenges, and the importance of relational communication and collective coping when a loved one begins to slip away irreversibly. Innovatively cowritten with an Alzheimer's patient, this narrative tells of a woman wanting to live life fully and not be governed by a diagnosis, committing her life to care for others in her family with the disease, and speaking out as an advocate in the much broader and bigger fight for a cure. Together, these contributors speak of the power of family/relational memories, relationships, and the communication that helps to navigate the middles of life for the women featured in these chapters.

The third part of this book (Endings and Legacies) begins with a powerful narrative account of a mother's traumatic and life-changing health experience, by Leda Cooks, that highlights the need for personal and relationally grounded narrative approaches to health experiences (chapter 10: Sylvia's Story/the Story of Sylvia: Narrating the Personal and Relational in Patienthood). The next two chapters pair together around the communicative process and experience of women caring for those who once cared for them, whether between daughter and mother, chapter 11 by Deleasa Randall-Griffiths (Linked Lives: A Narrative Exploration of Positivity and Dialectic in a Patient's Experience) or between daughter and father, chapter 12 written by Deanna F. Womack (A Narrative Account of Father-Daughter Conversations Near the End of His Life). Both these chapters, in their own unique ways, show a central concern in the women's heath narratives of giving care back to a caregiver—life to a life-giver. Adapting one's life to the needs of another, commitment to loved ones through role reversal, being flexible, creative, resourceful, and even innovative, as situations and shifting needs and identities demand, and the deep meaning of poignant moments of caring connection and of loss, narrated across lifespans, shine inspiringly through these narratives. Finally, Spencer's chapter 13 (A Narrative Legacy of Family Caregiving) explores the brighter, and beautiful, legacy of family caregiving as it is passed on across generations of her family as her mother's health declines through Alzheimer's. This chapter illustrates how narratives are shared and inherited, and that they can also be treasures discovered and retold to makes sense of relational identities and lives after a mother is gone. Collectively, these chapters also push our understanding of "lifespan" past the notion of one individual life into patterns and cycles that span multiple generations of families. There are values, qualities, and positive practices of family and relational communication that can cut across individual lifespans and have more enduring and ongoing lifespans of their own.

Finally, a note on the cover design. The image, which is inspired by a moment in chapter 10 between a mother and daughter, poignantly captures much about each of the women's narrative of this book. Rather than implying a "battle" archetype to their health disruptions or illnesses—something none of them directly invoke, the image speaks of moments of togetherness, and (intergenerational) support, captured in the physical expression of strength, balance, mutuality, and flexibility. These are themes that all the women depicted in this book speak to and exemplify in their own personal and relational ways.

Part I

Beginnings

Chapter One

This Wasn't How the Story Was Supposed to Go

Navigating Unmet Expectations During High-Risk Pregnancies and Premature Birth

Jennifer Hall

Narratives are a unique form of communication that serve multiple functions at the intrapersonal and interpersonal and societal levels. Because we engage with and come to understand the world through stories (Fisher, 1984), they provide a way for individuals to make sense of their lived experiences, transform their identities, create connections with others, and establish and reinforce societal and cultural norms (Batt, 2007; Moran, Murphy, Frank, & Baezconde-Garbanati, 2013; Russell & Arthur, 2016). As people navigate their way through their lifespan, stories are one of the primary ways that they can learn about and develop expectations for what new experiences and phases of life will be like (Reese et al., 2011; Singer, 2004). When facing an unknown situation such as dealing with a medical condition, other's stories can serve as models for what these situations will be like. When it comes to decision-making, rather than relying on rational thought per se, Fisher argues that people use stories, both their own—and those they have encountered, to determine the best course of action.

Health disruptions and illness are often marked by uncertainty, and narratives can provide information about everything from likely symptoms to possible prognosis, as well as good ways through. Because narratives are central to the way we think about and experience the world (Hyden 1997), they are integral to how people understand and make sense of health and illness-related experiences (Frank, 1995; Sharf and Vanderford, 2002). One of the powerful things that narratives assist people in doing is to bring a sense of order to otherwise chaotic experiences. Pennebaker and Seagal explain that "once a complex event is put into a story format, it is simplified. The mind doesn't need to work as hard to bring structure and meaning to it" (1999, p. 1250). This chapter examines the various ways that narratives provide help to women experiencing difficult pregnancies.

NARRATING PREGNANCY AND CHILDBIRTH

Pregnancy and childbirth represent major life events and milestones that many women anticipate and experience. Therefore, it is not surprising, that in the realm of pregnancy and childbirth, narratives play key roles. At the individual level, women often create narratives as they look back on their experiences to reflect on them and make sense of what occurred (Callister, 2004). Narratives also play a role in assisting women in transforming into the mother role (Kruger 2003; Brubaker & Wright 2006). Navigating pregnancy can be difficult and stressful as women must make decisions about their prenatal care, medical procedures, and childbirth as well as negotiate their changing identities and relationships (Besser & Priel, 2003). When a woman experiences complications or traumatic events surrounding their pregnancy and birth, the sense-making role of narratives can be healing and cathartic (Beck, 2006). Sharing her story and making sense of the elements of the story that were traumatic and painful, can help a woman to integrate the problematic elements of their experiences into their broader life story in healthy ways. The act of creating a story after a traumatizing event can help individuals cope with and heal from the trauma (Gumb, 2018; Sewell & Williams, 2002; Lane, Meyers, Hill, & Lane, 2016).

Telling their stories can also connect women to other women who can provide much needed social support, particularly when they have had similar experiences (Callister 2004; Affonso, 1977). The social support that women can receive through sharing their story with others is an example of the power narratives can have in interpersonal and online settings. Sharing pregnancy and delivery stories can also create connection between the teller and the listener, providing a common link among women from all generations who have experienced pregnancy, labor, and birth (Barlett, 2001; Gould, 2017). At a broader level, stories become a way that societies and cultures frame lived experiences by defining various aspects of motherhood (Kerrick & Henry, 2017; Horstman, Anderson, & Keuhl, 2007). Individuals may not even realize that these prevailing narratives exist, as they are almost ubiquitous and show up in the stories others tell, on television, in books, and in movies. In the United States, although there has been some room for variation in the basic pregnancy and birth narrative, in terms of specifics of how a pregnancy proceeds and how a child is born remains quite consistent.

The multiple stories that women encounter relating to pregnancy and childbirth matter, because no story exists in isolation. As Fisher explains, the meaning and value of a story is always a matter of how it relates to and compares with other stories. Cottle (2002) explains that any encounter with another narrative constitutes an exchange or an interaction, as we always respond to a narrative either by commenting on the words of the other or by applying the other's narratives to our own. Frequently, the response to hearing another narrative is to invoke our own story and, in doing so, we can either affirm or negate another's tale. Additionally, as we reflect on the stories we hear, we can allow those stories to alter our own stories and worldview. Cottle states, "we tend to hear another's story with our own stories, our lenses, as it were, shaping and refining the content and tone of what we are encountering" (p. 535). Additionally, studies have found that women rely on stories they hear from others or consume from media as a primary source of information about pregnancy and birth (Frawley et al., 2014; Bessett & Murawsky, 2018).

When women's experiences, the emotions they are feeling, and the stories they construct about their experiences are vastly different from the stories they have heard, seen, or read, they may experience tensions within self when working to understand those differences. This chapter helps to answer the question of what happens when women's lived experiences do not match the stories they have encountered or the stories they have imagined for themselves about pregnancy, childbirth, and early motherhood. While narratives can be a source of healing and connection for women (MacLellan, 2015; Wasserman & Wasserman, 2017), is it possible that stories can also be a source of confusion, contradiction, and pain?

WOMEN'S NARRATIVES OF HIGH RISK PREGNANCY AND PREMATURE BIRTH

One of the reasons it is important to talk about the experience of high-risk pregnancy and premature birth is that it is so common. It is estimated that 6 to 8 percent of pregnancies in the United States are classified as high-risk each year (USF, 2018). The March of Dimes reported that in 2011, 1 in 8 infants in the United States was born prematurely, which is over 450,000 infants a year. Prematurity is defined as any gestation less than 37 weeks ("March of Dimes Peristats," 2014). The rate of preterm birth often surprises people, and it is still a puzzle to medical professionals as to why the rate in the United States remains so high as compared to other countries. Given our advanced medical system and women's access to prenatal care, it is somewhat of a mystery as to why the preterm birth rate in the United States is higher than developing countries such as Kenya, Ethiopia, and Sudan. Risk factors for premature birth include being pregnant with twins or higher-order multiples (Chism 1997), being older than thirty-five or younger than seventeen, medical conditions such as high blood pressure and diabetes, and incompetent cervix, as well as environmental factors including stress, physically demanding work conditions, and lack of prenatal care.

Infants born prior to 37 weeks are at risk of experiencing a host of complications including jaundice, apnea, an increased risk for infection due to an immature immune system, mental retardation, learning disabilities, cerebral palsy, and vision and hearing problems (March of Dimes, 2016). The earlier an infant is born, the more severe the complications and issues they face tend to be. Infants born earlier than 34 weeks are at an increased risk for respiratory distress syndrome caused by a lack of surfactant, brain bleeds that can cause brain damage, heart conditions, necrotizing enterocolitis (i.e., a life threatening intestinal problem), retinopathy of prematurity (ROP), which untreated can lead to vision loss, and Patent Ductus Arteriosus (PDA), a heart condition where the ducts in the heart do not close properly.

Because of their small size and underdeveloped body systems, most premature infants spend time in the NICU (neonatal intensive care unit). In addition to the many risks premature infants face for long-term complications, they also face immediate, life-threatening challenges. Premature infants lack an adequate amount of body fat to regulate their body temperatures, so they often need to be kept in a heated incubator or isolette. An underdeveloped sucking reflex as well as an immature digestive system can also lead to feeding issues. Finally, many premature infants need respiratory assistance as their lungs have not fully developed (March of Dimes, 2016). When women are confronted with fears of these medical issues during their pregnancies or these issues are the reality their premature infants are living, the question arises of how stories are serving as sources of either support and healing or of difficulty.

Method

Ninety-five women who experienced a high-risk pregnancy, premature labor, or premature birth participated in semi-structured interviews. The interviews consisted of questions about women's pregnancy experience, their labor and delivery, and their lives after their children were born. Participants experienced a wide array of medical conditions during pregnancy including quadruplet, triplet, and twin pregnancies, preeclampsia, diabetes, advanced maternal age, placenta previa, an incompetent cervix, HELPP syndrome (a variant of preeclampsia), and PROM (premature rupture of membranes). Some women delivered early due to fetal distress such as IUGR (intrauterine growth restriction) while other women simply went into premature labor that could not be stopped. More than half of the participants had dealt with some type of infertility and undergone fertility treatments to achieve pregnancy. Participants delivered their children between 18 and 38 weeks and their children spent between 0 and 235 days in the NICU. Through qualitative analysis and careful rereading of the transcripts using ground theory and the constant comparison method (Glaser & Strauss, 1967), representative and exemplar narratives of women's experiences were highlighted. Participants were given the option to use a pseudonym or their own name.

The following narratives provide examples of women whose pregnancies and/or birth experiences were not typical or were not what they had expected. These examples illustrate how women interacted with, responded to, and used stories that they encountered as they navigated their ways through unknown and unanticipated experiences. Some of the themes that arose from the stories were the disruption a high-risk pregnancy created in the story women assumed they would live, the envy that some women felt when they encountered stories of uncomplicated pregnancies, and the grief that accompanied many women's stories.

The Pregnancy Experience: Exemplar Narratives

Based on what they had seen or heard or even experienced themselves during prior pregnancies, women had a set of expectations about what being pregnancy would be like. For most women, other than expecting some physical discomfort, women pregnant with only one infant with no other medical complications had generally positive ideas about how their pregnancies would progress. While they had heard stories or seen stories on TV of people who experienced pregnancy complications, for the most part, the stories they knew of pregnancy were those of uncomplicated pregnancies where a woman carried her baby to term. Additionally, women had clear ideas of how others would react to and celebrate their pregnancy and new child. Many talked about expecting showers, friendly comments from strangers, and general excitement from friends and family. When lived experiences did not fit with their expectations, many women had feelings of anger, bitterness, envy, and sadness that arose because of their unexpected circumstances, and these permeated their narration. An example of this can be found in Jen's story. As this mother of twins related her experience, she spoke openly about her struggle to reconcile her lived experience with her expectations.

At 15 weeks, Jen was placed on strict bed rest after her cervix started shortening. Because of her bedrest, she was unable to participate in many of the traditional rituals and customs that accompany a pregnancy in the United States. She described how difficult this was for her, "It's something I deal with a lot, I feel very sad about. You know, I remember going out shopping for maternity clothes early. I was still working, and I got big fast. Like I couldn't fit into any of my work clothes after eight weeks. And I was working on Wall Street, so I had to wear a suit. So, I went out and had to go to Anthony and Lock, which were the only reasonable maternity clothes for working women. You know, I spent hundreds of dollars on those maternity clothes and I was on bed rest shortly after I did that. . . . It is one of the things that causes me sadness. Like sometimes more than their NICU time. . . . But I rarely got to you know, go to the grocery store and have people be like, and you know, being able to walk around in cute little outfits and to be pregnant in the world." While she understood the reason that she had to be on bed rest and is very thankful that she was able hold off delivery until 28 weeks, her story reflects a deep sense of sadness and discontent with the difference between her actual experience and what she had anticipated.

Catt is another woman who struggled when she thought about the public aspects of her pregnancy she missed such as being seen in public or having a stranger comment on her pregnancy. Catt went on strict bed rest at 17 weeks after two of her triplets were diagnosed with twin-to-twin transfusion syndrome. Twin-to-twin transfusion syndrome is when identical twins share one placenta and one twin takes a greater share of the nutrients, which can cause harm to the other twin. Her twins' case was so severe that she actually lost one of the twins in utero around 24 weeks. She had a tremendous amount of grief and sadness over the loss of her daughter, but she also had a large amount of grief and sadness about the typical pregnancy activities such as wearing maternity clothes that she missed out on. She explained, "And the other thing. I had like two pairs of maternity pants and pair of maternity shorts. But you know, after seventeen weeks of being on bed rest, no one's going to see you. So you know, what's the point? . . . So I feel like I missed out on a lot."

Another ritual that was important to women that many missed out on, or could not fully enjoy, was a baby shower. Customarily, in the United States, a baby shower is held a month or two before the due date so expectant mothers can get the gear and clothing they need to be prepared for the new baby. Women who are hospitalized or on strict bed rest because of pregnancy complications are sometimes physically unable to attend the event. When a high-risk pregnancy results in preterm delivery, a baby's birth may be before the date of an already scheduled shower. Other women choose not to have a shower as the outcomes of their high-risk pregnancy feels too uncertain, and the thought of having gifts that would remain unused or need to be returned if the pregnancy did not end successfully was too much to deal with. Beth Anne lost her twin boys at 18 weeks when she delivered them early. Later, when pregnant with triplets, she refused to let her family host a shower or buy anything for the babies during her pregnancy. She had bought some things in preparation for her twin boys and returning unused baby items was one of the most difficult things she ever had to do, and she was not willing to put herself through that again. "There is nothing worse than returning unused baby items," she explained.

Monica's son was born at 28 weeks when her severe preeclampsia necessitated an emergency delivery. When he was a few weeks old, her baby shower took place. She hesitated about going, worried about being away from the hospital, but the nurses encouraged her to attend. She attended but found that it was nothing like she had imagined it would be. She was not pregnant, eagerly awaiting the birth of her first child. Instead, she found herself opening gifts and looking at the baby clothes and equipment wondering if her tiny and medically fragile son would make it out of the hospital and be able to use them. Some of the women interviewed had a shower after their babies came home from the NICU, and often their babies attended their own shower, something that felt strange to many women as the typical story of a baby shower in American culture is a party held before a baby is born.

Samantha's twin daughters were born at just 26 weeks. While they were still in the NICU her friends and family hosted a shower. She tried to enjoy herself, but the entire time she felt odd knowing that her babies were in the hospital, still not big and healthy enough to come home. Some guests brought their own young babies to the shower, and Samantha found herself feeling angry that the babies were there while her own daughters were still dependent on various machines to survive. Her premature delivery disrupted the traditional timeline of the story of a pregnancy and birth and it was difficult for her to accept the new order of events. Nicole never had a baby shower, and she got to the point where no longer attends baby showers as they are too emotional for her. She explains, "I can't go to baby showers. It is just so much of a reminder of what I did not get. That is because I was in the hospital and I felt like we can't do anything because what would happen if they die? At a shower everyone talking is so excited and the pregnant person says something about how they can't wait to deliver, and it is just too much."

Another experience that many women look forward to is feeling the baby kick or move inside. When women give birth just after their second trimester, they had limited time to feel the movement. Yvette, mother of twins, was hospitalized at 24 weeks when she went into preterm labor. For the next three weeks, doctors were able to hold off delivery in part through the administration of magnesium sulfate, a medication that slows contractions and slows the general movement and muscle tone of the mother and infants. There were so many things during her pregnancy that she felt she missed. "I don't think I can ever get over the NICU. You can't put into words that kind of loss and even though I have two beautiful children. It's a loss that I never felt them kick. I had an emergency C-section, no one was there." Unlike the story she had imagined, she never got to enjoy her pregnancy, share the delivery with her husband, or hold her newborns immediately after the birth.

Nicole delivered so early that she never felt them moving and kicking as she delivered her twin sons at just 25 weeks. When she compares her experiences with the stories other women share, she often struggles to relate as she delivered before her third trimester. She also found that people who did not understand how dangerous it was to give birth so early, and because of this made assumptions about what it was like. Once a woman commented to her that she was lucky to have only been pregnant for 25 weeks because she must not have gained too much weight and didn't have a lot to lose postpartum. Nicole was so shocked by the comment that she just turned and walked away, not sure how to respond. She told me, "I never got to feel the babies kick. We have one picture of me with a slight belly. You feel like you walk around with an asterisk." Her pregnancy was so different than a typical one, that she feels like her story is an outlier and does fit in with the general stories that people tell and want to hear.

Delivery and Birth: Exemplar Narratives

Another area where women had a lot of expectations surrounded the birth of their children. For first-time mothers, there was a lot of uncertainty about what labor and delivery would be like, so they leaned heavily on others' stories to get an idea of what would happen. Many anticipated having a vaginal delivery, even though nearly one-third of the deliveries in the United States are cesarean sections. Even if women had anticipated a C-section due to known complications, very few women were prepared for an emergency delivery. Most had imagined going through several hours of labor or having a scheduled C-section, but they had not considered the possibility that due to complications and threats to their own health or their infant's health that there would be fewer than thirty minutes between learning that they needed to deliver and the birth or their children.

Heather, for example, was hospitalized at 27 weeks due to heavy bleeding. A week later, her doctor determined that Heather's health was at risk and she needed to deliver immediately. It was the middle of the day, so Heather was alone at the hospital and her husband who worked almost an hour away did not have enough time to get there. Before going in to the OR, the nurses warned her that her daughter would most likely come out not breathing. She is incredibly thankful for the kind anesthesiologist who talked her through her incredibly frightening and stressful delivery but is also sad about how traumatic the experience was. Her delivery was nothing like the stories she had heard.

Sarah was admitted to the hospital at 25 weeks pregnant after it was discovered that she had almost no amniotic fluid and an ultrasound showed no fetal breathing. She mentally prepared herself for a long hospital stay, but two days later, nurses woke her up in the middle of the night and told her that her son Conner's heart rate had dropped dangerously low and she was being rushed to an emergency C-section. Up until this point she says she was in denial, never letting herself believe that her son would come so early. As the nurses talked to her, she kept telling them that it was too early and that she didn't understand why they were making her deliver him. She says her memory of the delivery is somewhat spotty, but she does remember shaking with fear and thinking that there were just so many people in the operating room. Immediately after Conner was born, a nurse held him up for Sarah to see and then quickly took him to be worked on by the medical team. Sarah does remember repeatedly telling anyone who was near that her son's name was Conner. "I really needed them to know his name," she explained, "because you can't ask baby X not to die." Fortunately, Conner survived and after a lengthy NICU stay he was able to come home.

Cora also recounted her story of a traumatic and unexpected delivery. At 29 weeks, Cora noticed that her daughter Lily had not been moving that day. This made her anxious, so she and her husband turned to Google and tried a variety of things to get the baby to move. When none of these worked they decided it was better to be safe than sorry, so they headed to the hospital to have things checked out. At the hospital, monitoring showed that they baby's heart was repeatedly dropping too low, so the doctor ordered an ultrasound and started to look for specific movements from the baby. After a few minutes, her medical team left the room to discuss their findings and Cora felt that something was very wrong. Just five minutes later a delivery team descended into her room and started to prep her for an emergency C-section. The news was so unexpected and terrifying that Cora had a hard time processing was happening. She explained, "I knew she was going to be so tiny, I just kept telling them I don't want to see her, I don't want to see her." In her work as a pediatric hospice social worker, Cora had known many premature children who had serious complications and disabilities. Her prior knowledge and experience meant that she knew the worst possible outcomes and had a hard time envisioning a positive one.

In the operating room, the anesthesiologist struggled to get the epidural in. He told her that time was critical because her baby was in great distress and if she was not delivered soon, she would die. After the epidural was in, the doctors rushed to get the baby out and Cora heard a tiny yelp, so she knew that at least Lily had been born alive, but this brought her little comfort. "I could see the look on the nurse's face," she told me, "and it was terrible." Lily did survive, but the first days of her life were very touch and go. This delivery was so far from what she expected that she still wakes up and has nightmares about it.

The differences between the expected stories and the reality frequently led to feelings of anger, bitterness, and envy. Marie, mother of triplets, talked about her feelings of resentment when she heard stories about other women's non-complicated pregnancies and births, "The way I view them is like, wow they have it so easy, they have a few contractions, they go in, they push a baby out, and they're holding their baby immediately, they're breastfeeding their baby, everything is fantastic, everybody is healthy and everybody goes home. They have people bring them cooked meals and everything is great." Marie described the typical and desired story that seems to be how most women experience pregnancy and birth. She explained how the story was different for women with a high-risk pregnancy, "For us it's like, you just have all of these different scares and all of these different worries, and you want all of your concerns to be addressed, but then you don't even want to think about it. You are just trying to stay positive. Then you have all this rush of hormones. Good grief! How do you deal with all of that? I don't know. I think it's a little different. You just have a lot more to think about than a normal pregnancy." She knew that any pregnancy, even those with no complication can be difficult and have traumatic aspects, but these other stories seemed so much easier than her own. The stories she had previously encountered shaped the story she told about her own pregnancy. Her story not only told about the things that had happened to her but also included elements of bitterness and longing as she consider how different her story was from the norm.

Neonatal Experiences: Exemplar Narratives

Another situation that women had expectations for was how they would spend the first moments of their infants' lives. Based on stories they had heard and what they had seen on TV, many women imagined getting to hold the baby immediately after delivery. Because of the precarious health of many of their babies, many mothers interviewed were only able to see a quick glimpse of their child or children before a medical team transported them to the NICU. Women talked about the grief and sadness they felt over missing out on what they saw as a pivotal life moment. Some felt almost embarrassed, but how sad they were as they rationally knew that their children had survived, but they still felt like something was missing.

Jana, who experienced two high-risk pregnancies, described how the stories around her had given her a set of expectations surrounding pregnancy and motherhood. She explained, "You know that you've seen the baby story or heard from your friends and you've seen the pictures of their blog in the hospital of them delivering the baby and holding the baby right away and being able to bond with the kid for that two day period." Like many of the women interviewed, Jana's actual births looked nothing like this picture.

Merillat was not only worried when her son was born eight weeks early, but she was also extremely upset that she and her son had to be separated immediately after he was born at 32 weeks, and she considered his birth a traumatic experience. Merillat went into labor at 32 weeks, and doctors were unable to stop the contractions, so her son was born six hours after her water broke. Her experience led her to start a support group for women who were separated from their children at birth either because of prematurity or other medical conditions. Three years after his birth, she still had a very strong emotional reaction to talking about what happened. She explained, "I think that from the time I started wanting to have children it was the one experience in life I could identify as being a spiritual experience, the carrying and bearing and raising of a child. I had read a lot about what happens in a woman's body. You give birth to your baby and, at the moment of the birth, this is the biggest rush of hormones you will ever have, and they put the baby on top of you and your eyes meet, and it is the indelible spiritual moment. I did not get that at all and he had to be taken away and I will never get over that."

Another moment that did not go the way that many women had expected was when they were finally able to go and visit their babies in the NICU for the first time. Jennifer had an emergency C-section at just 28 weeks and had to be put under for the surgery, so she did not see or hear her daughter before she went to the NICU. Her first visit to the NICU was completely overwhelming. She had seen a picture of her daughter and her husband had tried to prepare her for how small her daughter was but seeing her in person was still shocking. She told me, "I just wanted to hold her. I just felt awful like I failed her, and I couldn't hold her. I felt so awful and I wanted to say to her, this is not what I was supposed to do, and I was supposed to keep you in and you were supposed to come out healthy and happy." Her daughter was so small and fragile that it was three days before Jennifer could hold her and the entire time Jennifer just sat and cried and thought to herself, "This was not what it was supposed to be."

Another difficult day for many women was the day that they were discharged from the hospital while their baby or babies were still in the NICU. Leaving the hospital with a newborn was another moment that women had created a story for. They pictured being wheeled out of the hospital holding their baby while their husband or partner pulled up the car to the front door. Many women left the hospital in a wheelchair, but when they went outside without their baby it felt wrong as this was not how it was supposed to go. For women whose infants had long NICU stays, the feelings of the story not going how it was supposed to be continued as they tried to navigate life between the hospital and home.

Heather's daughter was born at 28 weeks after an ultrasound showed that the baby had stopped growing. Heather had two older children, so staying at the hospital long term was not an option. She lived forty-five minutes from the hospital, and with high gas prices, it was not economically feasible for her to go the hospital every day and there was no one at home to watch her other children while she was gone. As she drove away, knowing how hard it would be to come back and see her baby, she was absolutely devastated. She just kept thinking that mothers and babies were supposed to be together. In a very surprising and fortunate turn of events, Heather won a local raffle and the money was enough to cover her gas to and from the hospital each day. It was still a very stressful and difficult time for her as she was home with her kids all day and then would drive herself to the hospital through busy Las Vegas traffic each evening so that she could spend a few hours with her daughter. Her husband was working overtime, so he was not able to go to the hospital often and Heather was split between her world at home and her world in the NICU.

Sometimes because their story did not fit the norm, this made women want to have another child so that they could have the story they had imagined. Denise, mother of triplets, talked about what it was like for her after the chaos of the first year had passed. "Afterwards, when my kids were around two, I went through this phase where I really wanted to get pregnant again because I felt like I got gypped out of a pregnancy. You know, because I didn't get to wear maternity clothes. I wore like a T-shirt, my husband's 3X T-shirt. And you know, I didn't get to go out shopping and I didn't get to do all those things. So, I went through a lot, because my friends who had been through pregnancy I got to see them, you know, experience that. They got to take pregnancy exercise classes and all that and I didn't get to experience that. So, I went through a phase where I really wanted to be pregnant and wear cute little bib overalls and all that."

DISCUSSION AND CONCLUSION

The stories women told me about their high-risk pregnancies and the way they talked about their experiences revealed two things. First, the stories that women had previously encountered about pregnancy, childbirth, and early motherhood had a primary role in shaping women's expectations. Second, when a woman's lived experience did not meet those expectations, and the plot of her own story did not match that of the imagined story, many women struggled with how to make sense of and cope with this narrative gap. The challenge for women who experienced high-risk pregnancies, and those who support them, is to find a way to tell a story that recognizes and acknowledges the pain and trauma but does not cast the women's story as "wrong" in some way.

One way to help women is to provide access to multiple stories about motherhood and birth. In doing so, women may see elements of their own experience in other stories and feel less like their story is an aberration or abnormal. Exposure to other stories with more diverse plots can also help women create new expectations for what a high-risk pregnancy and premature delivery will be like. Stories about different paths to motherhood and parental bonding could also help women to cope with the stressful beginnings of their children's lives. For example McDermott-Perez (2007) presented the experiences of adoptive parents as a counternarrative to a commonly held belief that the first moments of life are a critical moment in terms of mother and child bonding as some physicians and child-rearing experts have argued (Spock and Needlman 2004). Many adoptive parents who are not present at the birth and may even adopt older children are strongly connected and bonded with their children despite not holding them immediately after birth. Stories such as these could help women to reframe their own thinking and their motherhood stories.

Due to the stories women consume from an early age, they often develop unrealistic expectations about what their pregnancy and birth experiences will be like. When preterm labor and premature birth occur, women's worlds are often turned upside down as the things they anticipated doing and feeling and saying, do not happen. While disappointment and grief often are natural, human reactions to situations like this, as no one wants to see their baby born sick, struggling to do basic things such as breathe and eat, women's sadness and grief is often compounded by the loss of the experiences they had imagined. Women must let go of their wishes for a perfect baby shower, holding their newborn, and bringing home their baby from the hospital with them. Additionally, when a baby is born early, most women find themselves in uncharted territory as they have no idea what it is like to parent a preemie, have a child in the NICU, and live with the constant anxiety that something will be seriously wrong with their child. Women can be helped if they have ways to enrich their narrative vocabularies to both cope with unmet expectations and to develop new expectations for what their experience will be like.

REFERENCES

Affonso, D. (1977). "'Missing Pieces'—A Study of Postpartum Feelings." *Birth* 4 (4): 159–64.
Barlett, J. R. (2001). "Older Women, Personal Narratives, and the Power of Sharing With Adolescent Girls." *Adultspan Journal*, 3(1), 32. Retrieved from http://search.ebscohost.com/login.aspx?direct=true&db=aph&AN=7678436&site=ehost-live
Batt, S. (2007). "Limits on Autonomy: Political Meta-Narratives and Health Stories in the Media." *American Journal of Bioethics*, 7(8), 23–25. https://doi.org/10.1080/15265160701462335.
Beck, C. (2006). "Pentadic Cartography: Mapping Birth Trauma Narratives." *Qualitative Health Research* 16 (4): 453–66.
Besser, A., & B. Priel. (2003). "Trait Vulnerability and Coping Strategies in the Tranistion to Motherhood." *Current Psychology* 15 (6): 57–72.
Bessett, D., & Murawsky, S. (2018). "'I guess I do have to take back what I said before, about television': pregnant women's understandings and use of televisual representations of childbearing." *Sociology of Health & Illness*, 40(3), 478–93. https://doi.org/10.1111/1467-9566.12658.

Brubaker, S., & C. Wright. (2006). "Identity Transformation and Family and Family Caregiving: Narratives of African American Teen Mothers." *Journal of Marriage and Family* 5: 1214–28.
Callister, L. C. (2004). "Making Meaning: Women's Birth Narratives." *Journal of Obstetric, Gynecologic, and Neonatal Nursing* 33 (4): 508–18. doi:10.1177/0884217504266898.
Chism, D. (1997). *The High-Risk Pregnancy Sourcebook*. Los Angeles, CA: Lowell House.
Cottle, T. (2002). "On Narratives and the Sense of Sef." *Qualitative Inquiry* 8 (5): 535–49.
Fisher, W. (1984). "Narration as Human Communication Paradigm: The Case of Public Moral Argument." *Communication Monographs* 51: 1–22.
———. (1985). "The Narrative Paradigm: An Elaboration." *Communication Monographs* 52: 347–67.
———. (1989). "Carifying the Narrative Paradigm." *Communication Monographs* 56: 55–58.
Frank, A. (1995). *The Wounded Storyteller*. Chicago, IL: The University of Chicago Press.
Frawley, J., Adams, J., Broom, A., Steel, A., Gallois, C., & Sibbritt, D. (2014). "Majority of Women Are Influenced by Nonprofessional Information Sources When Deciding to Consult a Complementary and Alternative Medicine Practitioner During Pregnancy." *Journal of Alternative & Complementary Medicine*, 20(7), 571–577. https://doi.org/10.1089/acm.2014.0028.
Glaser, B. G., & Strauss, A. L. (1967). *The Discovery of Grounded Theory: Strategies for Qualitative Research*. Chicago: Aldine Publishing Company.
Gould, J. (2017). "Storytelling in midwifery: Is it time to value our oral tradition?" *British Journal of Midwifery*, 25(1), 41–45. https://doi.org/10.12968/bjom.2017.25.1.41.
Gumb, L. (2018). "Trauma and Recovery: Finding the Ordinary Hero in Fictional Recovery Narratives." *Journal Of Humanistic Psychology*, 58(4), 460–474. doi:10.1177/0022167817749703.
Hyden, L. (1997). "Illness and Narrative." *Sociology of Health and Illness* 19 (1): 48–69.
Horstman, H. K., Anderson, J., & Kuehl, R. A. (2017). "Communicatively Making Sense of Doulas within the U.S. Master Birth Narrative: Doulas as Liminal Characters." *Health Communication*, 32(12), 1510–1519. https://doi.org/10.1080/10410236.2016.1234537.
Kerrick, M., & Henry, R. (2017). "'Totally in Love': Evidence of a Master Narrative for How New Mothers Should Feel About Their Babies." *Sex Roles*, 76(1–2), 1–16. https://doi.org/10.1007/s11199-016-0666-2.
Kruger, L.-M. (2003). "Narrating Motherhood: The Transformative Potential of Individual Stories." *South African Journl of Psychology* 33 (4): 198–204.
Lane, W. D., Myers, K. J., Hill, M. C., & Lane, D. E. (2016). "Utilizing Narrative Methodology in Trauma Treatment with Haitian Earthquake Survivors." *Journal Of Loss & Trauma*, 21(6), 560–574. doi:10.1080/15325024.2016.1159113.
MacLellan, J. (2015). "Healing identity by telling childbirth stories on the internet." *British Journal of Midwifery*, 23(7), 477–482. Retrieved from http://search.ebscohost.com/login.aspx?direct=true&db=aph&AN=103609990&site=ehost-live.
March of Dimes. (2016). https://www.marchofdimes.org/peristats/Peristats.aspx.
"March of Dimes Peristats." (2014). www.marchofdimes.com/Peristats.
McDermott-Perez, L. (2007). *Preemie Parents: Recovering from Bab's Premature Birth*. Westport, CT: Praeger.
Moran, M. B., Murphy, S. T., Frank, L. B., & Baezconde-Garbanati, L. (2013). "The Ability of Narrative Communication to Address Health-related Social Norms." *International Review of Social Research*, 3(2), 131–149. https://doi.org/10.1515/irsr-2013-0014.
Pennebaker, James W, and Janel D Seagal. (1999). "Forminy a Story: The Health Benefits of Narrative" 55 (10): 1243–54.
Reese, E., Haden, C. A., Baker-Ward, L., Bauer, P., Fivush, R., & Ornstein, P. A. (2011). "Coherence of Personal Narratives Across the Lifespan: A Multidimensional Model and Coding Method." *Journal of Cognition & Development*, 12(4), 424–462. https://doi.org/10.1080/15248372.2011.587854.
Russell, L. D., & Arthur, T. (2016). "'That's What "College Experience" is': Exploring Cultural Narratives and Descriptive Norms College Students Construct for Legitimizing Alcohol Use." *Health Communication*, 31(8), 917–925. https://doi.org/10.1080/10410236.2015

.1018700.
Sewell, K. W., & Williams, A. M. (2002). "Broken narratives: trauma, metaconstructive gaps, and the audience of psychotherapy." *Journal of Constructivist Psychology*, 15(3), 205–218. doi:10.1080/10720530290100442.
Sharf, B., and M. Vanderford. (2002). "Illness Narratives and the Social Construction of Health." In *Handbook of Health Communication*, edited by L. Harter, P. M. Japp, and C. Beck, 9–34. Mahwah, NJ: Lawrence Earlbaum.
Singer, J. A. (2004). "Narrative Identity and Meaning Making Across the Adult Lifespan: An Introduction." *Journal of Personality*, 72(3), 437–460. https://doi.org/10.1111/j.0022-3506.2004.00268.x.
Spock, B., and R. Needlman. (2004). *Dr. Spock's Baby and Child Care*. New York: Pocket Books.
USF. (2018). https://health.usf.edu/care/obgyn/services-specialties/mfm.
Wasserman, J. A., & Wasserman, R. N. (2017). "Commentary: Making Sense of Everett's Arrival: A Commentary on the Power of Birth Narratives." *Narrative Inquiry in Bioethics*, 7(3), 225–230. https://doi.org/10.1353/nib.2017.0070.

Chapter Two

Giving Birth in a Distant Land

Patienthood and Self-Transformation of Another Kind

Krista Calvin and Avinash Thombre

Giving birth and becoming a mother is often a profound and transforming physical, mental, and emotional experience (Panuthos, 1984). Major psychological and social changes occur from the time of pregnancy, to birth of the baby, to the postnatal period (Atkas & Aydin, 2018). Support of the mother and child is linked to early brain development and behavioral well-being. Support is further linked to the baby's development later, and their forming early relationships (Kobayashi et al., 2017). A mother's early bond with her unborn baby, and sensitive early caregiving, are important for the healthy development of the child (Brandon et al., 2009).

The birth of a baby is a complex and wonderful event. Many physical and emotional changes happen for the mother and the baby. Overall, women look back positively on the birth experience if they can relate it to their own ability and strength (internal factors) and a trustful and respectful relationship with the medical staff (external factors) (Karlström, Nystedt, & Hildingsson, 2015). A woman's sense of trust and support from the father of the child and close family is another key aspect of a positive birthing process (Bohren et al., 2017). The feeling of safety promoted by a supportive communication environment is essential for gaining control during birth, and for focusing on techniques that enables the women to effectively manage labor (Savage, 2006). However, what if these vital elements are missing, and a woman finds herself giving birth in an unfamiliar environment, without the kind of support she might normally expect?

This chapter is centered on an autoethnographic narrative of a mother's (Calvin) first experience giving birth, which occurred in Argentina in the fall of 2017 during a study abroad class. The first author gave birth to a baby girl while traveling abroad in an "alien land," where she could not speak the native language and had no familiar social support. She fought through labor complications and gave birth to her daughter during her fifth month of pregnancy. The narrative provides her experience of being in a foreign place while dealing with critical medical issues. Using a transformative experiences framework (Thombre & Rogers, 2009) as a theoretical lens to examine the lived realities of a patienthood experience, the chapter provides implications for engaging in positive intrapersonal, as well as interpersonal, communication, and managing cultural differences in a difficult health situation.[1]

HEALTH NARRATIVE APPROACH

According to Berger and Luckmann (1966), we are constantly in the process of making sense of the world in which we reside through a process of social constructivism. Experiences and interactions with others help shape our sense of self and ideas of how to maintain a healthy lifestyle. Every individual has their own ideas and ways to cope with their health challenges or crises. Coping is the process of managing stressful situations (du Pre, 2017).

The term "narrative" derives from the Latin "narrare" (recounting) and "gnarus" (skillfully) (Price, 2011). Each of us create narratives for ourselves—stories that help us give meaning to our experiences. These may help us make sense of often ambiguous and difficult health experiences as well as shape our experiences and how we remember and share them (Mallick & Watts, 2007; Taylor, 2003; Sawyer, 2011). However, narratives are not simple and unproblematic because they are communicative phenomena (Caughlin et al., 2011). For the individuals who share their stories, narratives change and may develop incrementally, sometimes making it difficult for the listener to take stock of what they think. The narrator may have significant doubts about how others might receive their narrative (Schultz & Flasher, 2011). Listeners may welcome the story but also may judge the storyteller (for example, "is this the story of a 'good mother?'"). Schultz and Flasher (2011) further found that individuals are challenged every moment to make sense of our existence and to piece together what we have, and others have, or are doing. Every interaction represents a complex set of activities that include: striving to make sense of my situation, interrogation of what others are doing, and examination of what we are doing together (Caughlin et al., 2011).

Studies show the therapeutic effects of the use of narratives in healthcare, on both the listener and the teller (Epston & White, 1990). Studying patients' narratives is important for healthcare practitioners since it reveals their suffering in managing their illness and how they become resourceful about their condition (Freedman & Combs, 1996; Monk, 1997). Narrative methods can also elicit useful information from informants and serve as a vehicle for communicating the complex substance of their research to readers (Young, 1987). Put simply, narratives can provide access to patients' life worlds, connecting suffering to the webs of meanings, cultural conventions, and social relations within which suffering unfolds and is understood.

The health narrative approach distinguishes disease from illness (White, 2007). For physicians, disease refers to the disorders of the body; illness, however, is "how patients experience, perceive and live with a disease" personally and within the wider social network (Mirivel & Thombre 2010, p. 234). Further, Mirivel and Thombre (2010) found that surviving is first and foremost a communicative accomplishment. They concluded this by studying online social support exchanged among a group of burn survivors. Social support is integral. It does not just consist of statements of sympathy offered in response to a post/thread, but it also includes helpful and constructive advice, which reflect different perspectives on an experience. Thus, narratives are crucial both for the individual narrating and the listener by enabling each to make sense of an experience. The next section discusses transformation and how it can eventually lead to a change of perspective.

Theory of Transformative Experiences

Stories are a potent means of changing health-related attitudes, beliefs, and behavior because of recipients' transportation into the world of the narrative. Gerrig (1993) states that a narrative serves to "transport an experience away from the here and now" (p. 3), like feeling lost in a novel or a story—in a good way. Transportation leads to transformation, "a self-communicative experience that changes an individual's life so that priorities and self-identity are refocused" (Mohamed & Thombre, 2005, p. 347).

Using a metaphor of transportation highlights a cognitive process that leads to transformation of perceptions. In their study of online HIV stories, Mohammed and Thombre (2005) mention that individuals are likely to engage in a process of actively thinking about what could have happened to change an outcome. As a result, their perceptions are altered by the experience. The authors elaborate using Rogers' (2003) definition of transportation as "one can be transported by a narrative to another time and place by moving into an imagined situation" (p. 349). It involves motivating an individual's information search on a health topic starting from self-communication within an individual to a process of gradual realization that gears toward positive behavior change.

A transformative experience, as defined by Thombre and Rogers (2009), at its core involves an event that initiates a process of self-communication within individuals and changes their lives to refocus their priorities and redefine their self-identity. When a certain life event happens, it instigates a process of trying to understand the underlying wisdom of that event. The process starts by restoring one's beliefs and values, examining the cultural environment that will presume certain understandings, and looking for individuals with the same dilemma and shared discontent. Then starts the search for options of coping, rebuilding the self, and learning new skills. New skills require practice and mastery to build confidence and reintegrate into one's life based on conditions dictated by the new perspectives. du Pre and Ray (2008) named those experiences as "transcendent experiences," which they define as episodes where people discover an "overarching meaning or supra-meaning within experiences that might seem unthinkable" (p.198). In other words, the experience of hardship creates something meaningful throughout the course of unexpected circumstances—if this is how the person narrates the experience.

Thombre and Rogers (2009) argue that there are five stages of transformative experiences: heightened sensitivity to life, openness to change, disclosure to others, the need for information, and sharing narrative experiences with others. The first stage is *heightened sensitivity to life*. Whenever a person undergoes and overcomes a health disruption or crisis, they feel a heightened sensitivity to life. They begin to see things through a different light. For example, they may feel like they were taking life for granted and start to step out of their comfort zones and do things they wouldn't do before, like taking that trip, asking a person out, or building that house.

The second stage is *openness to change*. This stage reflects a person's choice to change bad habits and replace them with good habits. A person who was "scared" or "at a near death experience" because of health issues may realize that it is time for change and be more open to it. For example, a lung cancer survivor may choose to stop smoking and incorporate healthier eating habits and exercise. The third stage is *disclosure to others*. It was found that some people need to reflect with other people to rationalize their experiences and that often leads to disclosing to others. For example, they may partake in counseling services or communicate with a friend.

The fourth stage is *need for information*. To positively transform through the health challenge, one needs to understand it. It is bad enough that the patient is facing a health challenge, but not understanding it will create negative experiences. A good doctor or caregiver will provide necessary information to the patient and allow them to ask questions that make them knowledgeable, build trust, and create a sense of comfort and peace with the situation. The final stage is *sharing narrative experiences with others to arrive at a new identity*. This stage allows patients to use their health challenge as a testimony and support to others who are experiencing similar health challenges. For example, social support groups and social media groups provide patients with the opportunity to share their experiences with others in a positive and meaningful way.

Every health challenge and transformative experience is unique to everyone. A significant amount of the time this manifests itself in diagnoses of traumatic, life-changing, or mortal illnesses. For example, psychologist Victor Frankl (1959) reflected on his time in a German concentration camp to arrive at a transformation which proclaimed that during suffering more horrific than most of us can imagine the prisoners still found a reason to value life and to be optimistic about the future. Although this example is one of the outliers as far as severity, it is common among those who are afflicted with long-term ailments to transform their negative experiences into something uplifting that can carry them through to a state of conscious reflective peace.

Others say that they have been able to lay old grievances to rest and have developed a heightened appreciation for nature and loved ones (du Pre & Ray, 2008). As further stated by du Pre and Ray, "transcendence is not denial of one's circumstances, but an awareness that those circumstances exist within the framework of something more meaningful than one might previously have imagined" (p. 103). Transformative experiences are a common phenomenon that most humans face at one point or another. Transformation theory explores the different stages that a person will often experience through life altering events. In the following paragraphs, we discuss how a birthing health challenge filled with anxiety for the first author led to a positive transformative experience.

A NARRATIVE OF GIVING BIRTH FAR FROM HOME

For many women, becoming a mother means their hopes and dreams have come true. They love feeling their baby move inside them. They feel a sense of achievement in giving birth. They love holding, touching, watching, and smelling their baby. However, giving birth is a physically and emotionally draining process. In a study by Ayers (2007) more negative than positive emotions were described during birth: primarily feeling scared, frightened, and upset. Among different strategies of coping, women acknowledged taking a fatalistic view and focusing on the present, concentrating on the baby. Memories of birth include not remembering parts of the birth and forgetting how bad it was.

No matter how the natural process unfolds, giving birth is challenging in every aspect of the word. Women reported more panic, anger, thoughts of death, mental defeat, and dissociation during birth; after birth, they reported fewer strategies that focused on the present, more painful memories, intrusive memories, and rumination (Ayers, 2007). In the following paragraphs, the first author narrates her journey of giving birth in a foreign land, examined through the lens of transformative experiences.

The Fear of Losing My Baby

After a twelve-hour nonstop flight from Atlanta to Buenos Aires, on the second day of my arrival in the city as part of a study abroad class, I felt okay and was excited to experience a new culture. Even though I was five months into my pregnancy, my doctor had given me the green light to travel and be in this study abroad class. I did feel good. But within the first twenty-four hours, after we visited the famous 9 de Julio Avenue and the Obelisco and walked around the picturesque Corrientes area, I started to develop contractions and had a sleepless first night. The next day I took some painkillers, and we headed to see the Casa Rosada or the Pink house, and as we sat to have lunch, I noticed bleeding. I was hurting a lot, and we called the local 911. It took more than half an hour for the police to show up and another half hour for the ambulance to come. It was decided that I must be rushed to the nearest public hospital. It took forever for the ambulance to reach the hospital, due to being caught in the local traffic.

I lay there on a hospital bed in a Buenos Aires public hospital, a place like nothing I've ever seen. All patients were arranged in a large open space separated in tiny cubicles. Two of us were in a very small space that left no room for privacy. Sharp pains had now been surging through me for a few hours since I was rushed from the quaint little deli in Buenos Aires. I was drowning in fear and uncertainty, not knowing whether my baby was going to be okay. It had been a few hours since I spotted light bleeding, and everything in my memory told me I was about to lose the little girl I'd been singing to every morning while I got dressed for school. I sat and stared at the chair next to my hospital bed unable to escape my thoughts. The chair was a green plastic chair that you would expect to see on a person's patio, not bedside at a hospital. In the center of it was a huge hole the size of a cantaloupe. The chair was just as incomplete as I was feeling and was, to me, a direct reflection of the inadequacy of the rest of the hospital.

In addition to the unfamiliar atmosphere, I was unable to communicate with almost everyone about my condition, outside of brief visits from an occasional translator. I was far from home without one single family member to hold my hand. This was not how I expected my first motherhood experience to go. It was at that moment that my overwhelming fear turned into pure regret. Why did I travel? Should I have known I could go into labor at only five months? I hadn't had one inclination that this would happen from my doctor or anyone else I consulted with. Was it something I ate? Was it the water? Did I walk too much? Questions flooded my mind, filling me with negative thoughts as I struggled to keep up positive appearances to onlookers. These experiences directly relate to heightened sensitivity to life and openness to change—the first two stages of the theory of transformative experiences.

After spending the night in this public hospital where they were not able to stop my contractions, I was taken to a private hospital that was better equipped to handle my situation. There was no avoiding it. I was told in broken English, my *babe* would have to be delivered. I was given an emergency C-section at one of the most exquisite hospitals I'd ever seen. My fragile baby was born weighing only 522 grams. I was able to see my baby fleetingly before I could understand what was going on, and she was taken to the NICU.

Communicating Without Language

Members of my study abroad class, my only support system in Argentina, left to return home, while I remained and picked up the pieces of an entirely new life. My hospital room appeared more like a hotel room. The décor in lounge areas were trimmed with gold. My husband had now been notified and was desperately trying to make his flight. He'd worked so hard to qualify for his military privilege of enlisting into officer training. He was scheduled to report in two days. I knew my situation was going to shatter that endeavor. Our lives were planned and very structured before my trip. One day changed our lives completely. I knew my husband wouldn't leave me in Argentina alone. He arrived a day after I delivered my baby girl, and I felt comforted having family with me. Neither of us knew Spanish, and there was practically no one at the hospital who spoke English fluently.

We felt lost, having no idea what was going on most of the time. Our little baby girl was hooked up to a bunch of tubes and was given oxygen to help her breathing so that she could gain weight. Our sole comfort was in knowing that our little girl was still alive. Our communication with everyone became much like a constant game of charades consisting of sign language. There were long notes placed in my room that consisted of what I'm sure was important information if I could understand it. My nurses gave me medicine constantly. I had no idea what it was, but it was too difficult to try and communicate, so I just took it. *My* health wasn't what I was concerned about.

I longed for any moment that someone could give me information regarding my baby that I could understand. We used translator applications on our cell phones that proved to be only good with small talk and not good at all during real-time communication. Visual information became my primary form of gathering information. I could see my daughter's translucent skin and her tiny frame. I could see her draped in tubes with needles in her veins. I could see the numbers on machines and figure out which one was oxygen and which one measured her heartbeat. I could see her fingers turn black due to poor blood circulation, while the days passed one by one. After three weeks of despair and denial, I slowly accepted the situation that I was in. The things that I underwent correlate to the second and third stages of the theory

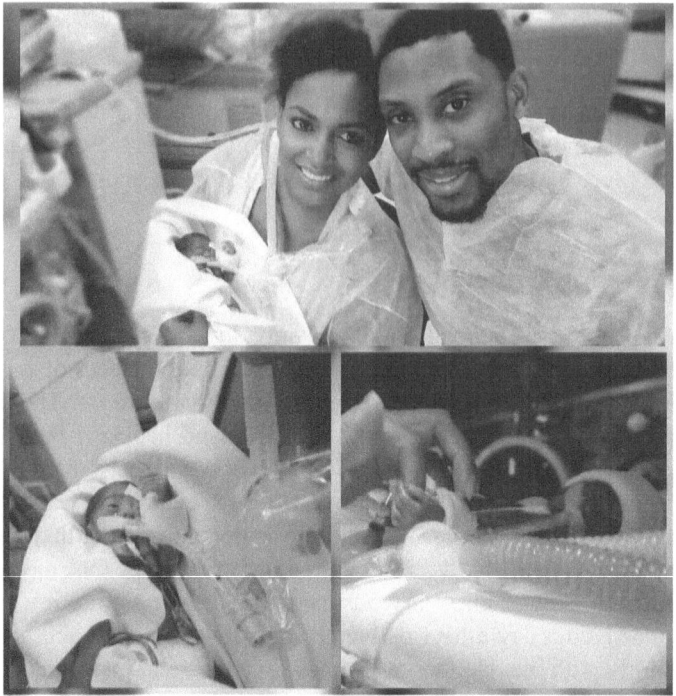

Figure 2.1. Birth of the baby and arrival of my husband Terrance Calvin. Photo courtesy of Krista Calvin.

of transformative experience, respectively, heightened sensitivity to life and openness of change.

I could see the hard work the medical staff was doing to care for our baby. I could see the culture of cheek kisses from males and females, so I understood that this was just as common as a kind pat on the back or a hug. I adopted this form of culture due to my observance of what it signifies. I learned key words in Spanish and Italian that are used constantly here and that I have to say regularly throughout my day in casual interactions. Some words in English that I had to learn the Spanish versions of are: hello, excuse me, can I see Kara, thank you, bye, fine, here, and beautiful (*hola, disculpe, puedo ver Kara, gracias, adios, multa, aqui, hermosa*). Knowing your numbers for exchanging money is extremely important as well, to avoid confusion when purchasing goods or services.

Maintaining Positivity

It is hard to maintain positivity when the apple of your eye is struggling to breathe. There were several nurses that cared for my daughter, Kara, but there was one who handled her a bit roughly. She was the oldest of the nurses. I sometimes turned down the opportunity to hold my baby when this nurse was present, because of how rough she was with her. She did not speak English and I feared that trying to talk to her about it could cause her to mistreat my baby. Instead, I tried a different form a communication with her, flattery. I learned a few words to try and build a bond with her and hopefully get her to feel more connected to my daughter. I thought that perhaps if I connect with her, she wouldn't see my baby as just another patient and treat her a little better.

There was one doctor who was there early in the morning that spoke decent English, so I was there every morning to ask her for an update. There was one question she asked me from time to time that always caught me by surprise, but it made me feel wonderful when asked. That question was, "How are *you* doing?" She focused on me for a moment, and although my world revolved around my beautiful baby girl, I found myself lost in gratitude that someone paused to acknowledge how I was feeling.

There was one situation where I needed new bottles so that I could provide milk for my baby. I was supposed to turn in milk and receive new bottles multiple times daily at a little office on the NICU floor. There were times I visited the pick-up office in the hospital, but no one was there. I was frustrated because my baby needed my milk and no one was ever there. Finally, I showed up while someone was there. I showed her my old bottles and awaited new ones. Instead of handing me new bottles, she closed the office door in my face. Frustrated, I started crying and threw the bottles in the used container as I stomped off. It was my fourth time walking several blocks to the hospital that day. I was still in pain from my own surgery, but I'd walk miles if it could help my baby. I felt helpless. My milk was the only thing I felt I could do for my baby, and here I was, helpless to get it to her because they wouldn't give me fresh bottles. This lady was standing in a room with a ton of them. All she had to do was hand me one, but she closed the door in my face. She came and found me about five minutes later and handed me some fresh bottles to use. She went on talking to me for about four minutes in Spanish. I did not understand one thing she said but I noticed she kept pointing at her wrist. Still fighting with my tears, I really just wanted her to leave me at the moment.

It was a week later that I decided to take a picture of a sign on a wall in our milk room and have a girl I'd met translate it. It was then, I learned the very specific hours that mothers are supposed to exchange milk bottles. Most of the assistants would just get me bottles regardless of the time, but no one went to the trouble of trying to help me understand the hours of operation in my language. My communication with this woman then became very positive. From then on, we tried to communicate with each other slowly as we taught each other new words from time to time. We both had to be open to each other's perspectives to foster better communication. Again, my experiences manifest the need for information—the fourth stage of theory of transformative experience. Again, I underwent the need to share information with others, which is the fifth stage of the theory of transformative experience.

Being Open at Every Stage and Utilizing Social Media

Self-disclosing information about my experience became a source of therapy for me. Social media was one of the things that remained familiar to me while I was stranded away from home. It was my lifeline to the things and people I knew. I found myself experiencing so many different emotions throughout my journey. Social media provided the support I needed to ensure my emotions were validated. If others knew what I was experiencing, would they understand? They did. Thousands of messages poured in from people offering supportive words of encouragement. I found myself logging on every chance I could to offer updates on the health of my baby and myself. If it took me longer than usual, people would start asking for the latest update. Strangers and friends walked with me through every stage of our journey.

Despite the haphazard connectivity of the internet and at times frustrating mobile phone issues, my husband and I shared every minute detail of the day-to-day happenings in the hospital with folks back home; our challenges with insurance, at times hilarious verbal and nonverbal communication with Argentinians, day-to-day activities of going around living life in an unknown city, cultural episodes, and much more. This open disclosure not only allowed an avenue for me to maintain sanity but also was an avenue for not keeping things bottled up inside me. This was happening almost unconsciously. Using social media proved to be very helpful in coping with what was a traumatic situation.

However, openly sharing my emotions on social media left me vulnerable to ridicule. Some people openly blamed me for traveling during my fifth month of pregnancy. It didn't matter that I was cleared to travel by multiple doctors. They took the position that I was wrong and deserved all the issues I was dealing with. Feeling attacked, I constantly defended myself initially, before realizing this behavior wasn't healthy for me. I found myself focusing on the handful of negative people rather than the thousands of supporters that offered positive encouragement. I learned to maintain my sense of self the hard way.

I interacted with the people on social media who genuinely cared. We created a GoFundMe drive asking for financial help. Hundreds donated, wanting to help with expenses without me even personally asking. I shared progress pictures on Facebook and Instagram of my little baby fighting for her life. I felt stronger when I shared. Thousands of people offering prayers gave me hope. Inside I felt that there was no way the God I serve wouldn't hear so many of us pleading for our dear baby Kara. The advice people offered truly helped me get through the tough times. I remember one of the most important messages I received which simply said, "It's okay to cry." I cried multiple times throughout the day, each day.

Forming New Relationships

As my story grew, so did the support of those it touched, including the local expat (American) community. Even while in a foreign country, God attracted all the right people into our lives as a way of saying, "I have not left you, and I have not forsaken you." The word of our precarious situation spread in the expat community and we were approached by a group of English speaking individuals. This beautiful group immediately accepted us as if we were family, eager to help in any way possible. Even when just spreading the news about our hardships and struggle with insurance issues, they were plenty helpful. We sent constant messages that we are doing okay. Kara has a support system in Argentina now as well. We will all continue fighting for what's right, while our little princess grows healthy and strong.

One young lady, who I had never ever met in person, contacted me about a social group that had been formed for expats in Buenos Aires. It was a group of English speaking foreigners that found themselves in Argentina for various reasons. I cried tears of joy as the group welcomed me after adding me to their WhatsApp group. They immediately arranged for a group dinner where my husband and I were the guests of honor. My husband and I were emotionally worn down from losing our stability, adapting to so much change, and only having each other to talk to. Finding a person or two would have been a delight. This was a group of more than thirty people willing to help us any way they could.

One person even offered their home as a place to stay without knowing anything other than our story. I felt more support from this group of strangers than my own family. They were absolutely amazing! They taught us basic aspects of navigating the day-to-day life: how to catch the subway, how to ride the bus, and which neighborhoods not to go to. They translated whenever possible so that we wouldn't have to spend money on translators. Not only did this experience make me grateful for becoming a part of this group, but it opened my heart to foreign situations in my own country. I found myself wanting to help where I could once I returned to North America. This group became so much more than just a support group. We were family: a family of foreigners in a distant land with nothing but positivity and encouragement to share with our members. The information and narrative sharing with others supported the transformative experience that I personally underwent.

Orienting to a New Survivor Self-Identity

Going through these changes made me a better person. I became a better wife as I leaned on my husband for emotional support as well as supported him through his tough moments. I became a strong mom. I watched my baby show amazing strength day after day as she gained weight, literally a few grams a day. I oscillated on this day-to-day roller coaster, happy if my baby opened her eyes for a brief time. Other days when she struggled to breathe and became blue, I felt overwhelmed. I had to be stronger during her surgery days and days she experienced medical issues. I knew she needed extra strength on those days. I was there with her every step of the way, singing to her as I fought back my own personal desire to break out in tears. I became protective as I thought of her future and all the people she would encounter. I became a more spiritual being. I prayed and meditated constantly to keep positivity in my mind.

I became more understanding of people who are different from myself. I matured. I liked who I'd become. I loved it, although it came with a greater sense of sensitivity and vulnerability. My priorities were getting my family home safely. At the forefront of every activity I tried to explore while in Argentina during my downtime, my thoughts were always on wanting to be

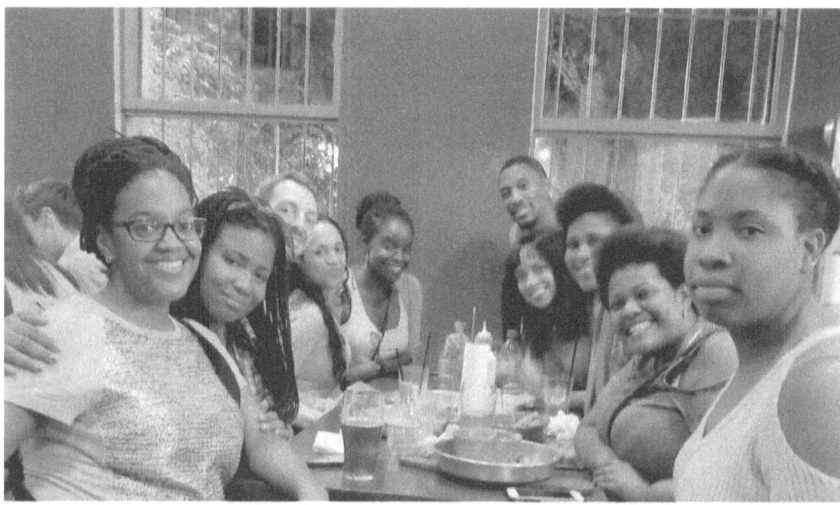

Figure 2.2. Our new friends in Argentina—forming usual social networks. Photo courtesy of Krista Calvin.

home. My relationship with my husband became more of a priority because I knew one day my daughter would learn communication by watching how we communicate with each other. I walked to the hospital three to five times a day to give her milk because it was one of the only things I could do for a while to contribute to her health.

My health became a priority because her nourishment came from my milk. My mental health was a priority because I couldn't allow myself to bring any negative emotion into her space. I was willing to do whatever I needed for my family even if it meant selling my house to ensure our stability while we couldn't work. Material possessions were nothing but tools to help what really mattered, my family. The last stage of theory of transformative experience talks about arriving at a new self-identity. My new survivor identity helped me to be there for my baby, myself, and my husband. Finally, after more than four months of constant struggle, my baby gained enough weight that she could breathe on her own and the doctors allowed us to get on the long, twelve-hour, nonstop flight back home.

RECOMMENDATIONS

During the first author's experience of delivering her baby and staying in the hospital for over four months, due to cultural and language barriers, the doctors rarely provided an explanation for the baby's condition. However, the first author consciously chose to focus on the positive outcomes and educate herself about her baby's condition. At the early stages, she realized a need for self-examination and to develop a course of action. This involves assessing the problem to decide which problem-solving techniques are needed. In addition, a lot of emotional adjustment was required for her to regain a sense of normalcy to move forward. As we examine the present patienthood narrative, a few reflections and associated recommendations come to our mind.

A Need for Personal Self-Examination

Concrete behaviors and new meanings emerge as individuals seek information and look for better management of their lives (Thombre & Rogers, 2009). The ambiguity that characterized the first author's health situation offered no choices but to stay strong and communicate to oneself about alternatives. Her decision to share her situation with others in the same situation, amid the uncertainties she felt, helped her appreciate the support while acknowledging her fears. Examining her own condition in the light of problems around her and her child helped her put into perspective the overall situation: the first step toward positive self-transformation. The present patienthood narrative supports the idea that individuals who come out as survivors

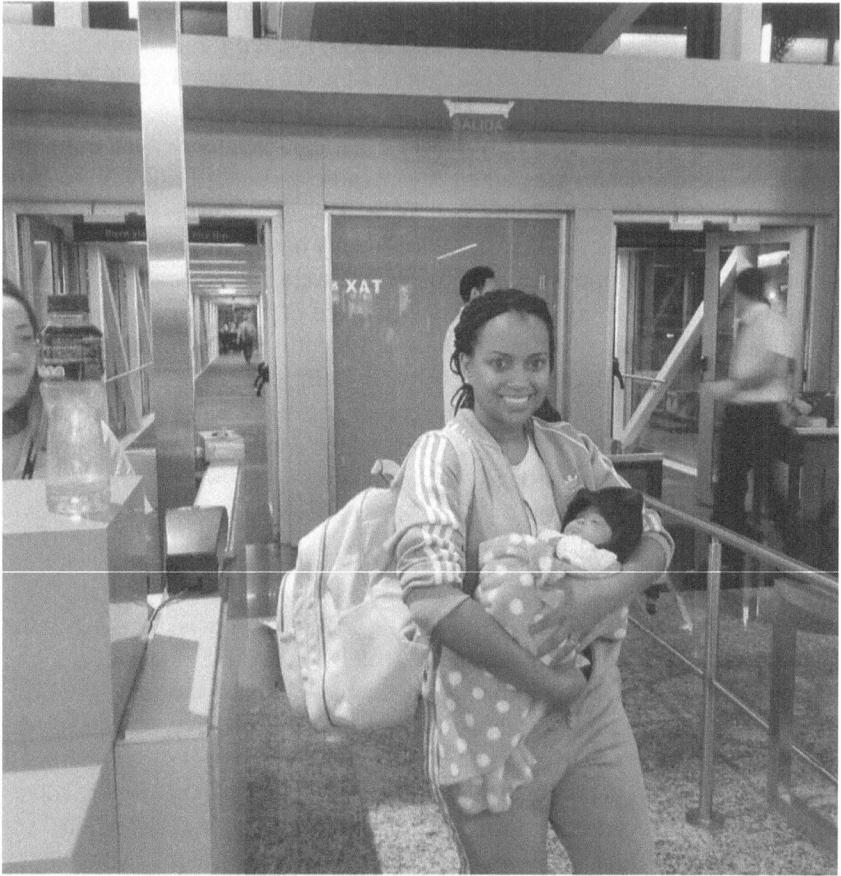

Figure 2.3. Leaving the hospital in Argentina to get back home. Photo courtesy of Krista Calvin.

of personal health tragedies need to undertake steps toward self-examination of their situation and engage in an intrapersonal dialogue with themselves that steers them toward transformation. While we acknowledge that it is challenging to engage in self-examination while undergoing disruptive situations, it nevertheless is important to experience this. The next step is developing a course of action.

Developing a Course of Action

After undergoing self-examination, according to Thombre and Rogers (2009), patients strive to gain control over their new situation, and as they do that, they engage in developing a course of action. The first step in this process is gathering information and understanding alternatives and precautions. For example, the first author joined groups on Facebook to ask others who had preemie babies with similar or worse conditions questions and started to identify with their situation. Second, patients start to change after sufficient information is collected. For example, as the first author read more about learning Spanish, she engaged in group discussions and became more assertive during follow up visits. This helped her realize the need for management of her baby's situation rather than a cure.

Third, patients adjust to new life styles. The first author had to develop a rigorous health plan for her baby to enhance weight gain for her baby. She adjusted to just being positive in an overtly negative situation that was beyond her control. Following the doctors' directions was a must. The fourth stage is reflection about the meaning of life and assessing emotional psychological options. She eliminated unessential distractions to attend often to her own personal and spiritual health needs. She had to rethink her priorities, which gave her a sense of self-efficacy and self-control. The fifth and final stage of the transformative process is developing a new identity. As she gained more insights into her baby's condition she was better able to manage her health and move forward considering the new adjustments.

Social Support and Coping

The suddenness of the event left the first author with much despair. Seeking emotional support, she always sought explanations behind her baby's condition and illness from doctors. In addition, she was offered a lot of help from the family of friends from the United States, and she formed a local support group consisting of Argentine Americans who organized a carpool and other necessary things for her, and prepared dinner during the early days after her hospital stay. Trying to educate herself about her baby's condition initiated a sense of empowerment as she learned that 50 percent of premature babies take a long time to gain weight and don't experience a lot of ups and down during this process. Thus, she was able to adjust her expectations and think about her choices. As she shared her story with others who had the same situation, she was grateful that her baby didn't develop any of the other complications. She even shared her experience with those who were first-timers. She concluded that everything was predetermined by God's will. God also wanted her to continue to do her best, and therefore, provided more opportunities over time. The social support with, and to, others became an important element in the process of the self-transformation she experienced.

CONCLUSION

In this chapter, we showed that undergoing patienthood in difficult circumstances triggers a process of self-reflection and developing a new identity, which eventually leads to transformation. Based on narrative reflection of the birthing process undergone by the first author, the following key communication strategies are identified. First, patients should be encouraged to disclose their own narratives on illness and how it affects their lives. In turn, caregivers should be able to provide comprehensive feedback that empowers patients and change their perspective towards disruption/illness. Second, having a strong social network of friends, professionals, or virtual communities is often "life enhancing" (du Pre, 2017, p. 210). Patients should be encouraged to voice their concerns so they can develop self-help skills and gain a greater sense of autonomy. Many patients do not experience effective transformative experiences. Some patients may drop out of treatment plans due to the absence of communication efforts and/or presence of cultural misconceptions. Therefore, caregivers are required to encourage patients to develop habits of self-care and efficacy, which enhances the healing process.

Finally, we assert that everybody has her or his own unique health challenges. Whether it is mentally, physically, extreme, or mild cases, they are all important and can all result in a positive transformative process with the right knowledge and action. Health challenges are unique to each individual and can positively influence the self and others through the transformative process.

NOTE

1. Acknowledgments: We would like to thank Dr. April Chatham-Carpenter for her continuous encouragement throughout the writing process. Also, profound thanks to Maria Sol Galli and her team at Universidad de Buenos Aires for providing vital support for the mother and baby. This piece is dedicated to the memory of Mr. Murlidhar Thombre (father of second author) who passed away in 2016.

REFERENCES

Aktas, S., & Aydin, R. (2018). The analysis of negative birth experiences of mothers: A qualitative study. *Journal of Reproductive Infant Psychology. 1*, 17. doi: 10.1080/02646838.2018.1540863.

Ayers, S. (2007). Thoughts and Emotions During Traumatic Birth: A Qualitative Study. *Birth: Issues in prenatal care. 34*, 3, 253–63. https://doi.org/10.1111/j.1523-536X.2007.00178.x.

Baruch, G. (1981). Moral tales: parents' stories of encounters with the health professions. *Sociology of Health and Illness*, 3, 3, pp. 275–96.

Berger, P. L. and Luckmann, T. (1966). *The Social Construction of Reality: A Treatise in the Sociology of Knowledge.* Doubleday & Company, New York.

Bohren, M. A., Hofmeyr, G. J., Sakala, C., Fukuzawa, R. K., & Cuthbert, A. (2017). Continuous support for women during childbirth. 6, 7, *Cochrane Database Syst Rev. doi:* 10.1002/14651858.CD003766.pub6.
Brandon, A. R., Pitts, S., Denton, W. H., Stringer, C. A., Evans, H. M. (2009). A history of the theory of prenatal attachment. *Journal of Prenatal Perinatal Psychology Health. 23*, 4, 201–22.
Caughlin, J., Mikucki-Enyart, S., Middleton, A., Stone, A. and Brown, L. (2011). Being open without talking about it: a rhetorical/normative approach to understanding topic avoidance in families after a lung cancer diagnosis. *Communication Monographs, 78*, 4, 409–36.
du Pre, A., & Ray, E. B. (2008). Comforting episodes: Transcendent experiences of cancer survivors. In L. Sparks, H. D. O'Hair, & G. L. Kreps (Eds.) *Cancer, communication and aging* (pp. 99–114). Cresskill, NJ: Hampton Press.
du Pre, A. (2017). *Communicating about health: current issues and perspectives*. New York: Oxford University Press.
Egbert, N., Sparks, L., Kreps, G. L., & du Pre, A. (2008). Finding meaning in the journey: Methods of spiritual coping for aging patients with cancer. In L. Sparks, H. D. O'Hair, & G. L. Keeps (Eds.), *Cancer, communication and aging* (pp. 277–91). Cresskill, NJ: Hampton Press.
Epston, D. & White, M. (1990). Story, knowledge, power. In Epston, D. & White, M., (Eds.) *Narrative means to therapeutic ends*. New York: Norton.
Frankl, V. E. (1959). *Man's search for meeting*. Boston: Beacon Press.
Freedman, J. & Combs, G. (1996). Shifting paradigms: From systems to stories. In Freedman, J. & Combs, G. *Narrative therapy: The social construction of preferred realities*. New York: Norton.
Gebbers, T., de Wit, J. B. F., & Appel, M. (2017). Transportation into narrative worlds and the motivation to change health-related behavior. *International Journal of Communication, 11,* 486–906.
Gerrig, R. J. (1993). *Experiencing narrative worlds: On the psychological activities of reading*. New Haven, CT: Yale University Press.
Handford, P. (2000). *The Curtis method of childbirth education*. Retrieved from https://curtismethod.com/quotes/90/.
Karlström, A., Nystedt, A., & Hildingsson, I. (2015). The meaning of a very positive birth experience: focus groups discussions with women. *BMC Pregnancy and Childbirth, 15*, 251. http://doi.org/10.1186/s12884-015-0683-0.
Kobayashi, S., Hanada, N., Matsuzaki, M., Takehara, K., Ota, E., Sasaki, H., Nagata, C., & Mori, R. (2017). Assessment and support during early labour for improving birth outcomes. *Cochrane Database Syst Rev. 20*, 4. doi: 10.1002/14651858.CD011516.
Mallick, J. & Watts, M. (2007). Personal construct theory and constructivist drug education. *Drug and Alcohol Review, 26*, 595–603.
Mirivel, J. C., & Thombre, A. (2010). Surviving online: An analysis of how burn survivors recover from life crisis. *Southern Journal of Communication, 75*, 1–23.
Mohammed, S., & Thombre, A. (2005). HIV/AIDS stories on the World Wide Web and transformative experiences. *Journal of Health Communication, 10*, 4, 347–60.
Monk, G. (1997). How narrative theory works. In G. Monk., Winslade, J., & Crocket, K. (Eds.,) *Narrative therapy in practice: The archeology of hope*. Jossey Bass: San Francisco, CA.
Panuthos, C. (1984). *Transformation through birth: A woman's guide*. Santa Barbara, CA: Praeger.
Placksin, S. (2000). *Mothering the new mother: Women's feeling and needs after childbirth, a resource guide*. New York: Newmarket Press.
Price, B. (2011). Making better use of older people's narratives. *Nursing Older People, 23*, 6, 31–37.
Rogers, E. M. (2003, 5th edition). *Diffusion of innovations*. New York: The Free Press.
Savage, J. S. (2006). The lived experience of knowing in childbirth. *Journal of Perinatal Education. 15*, 3, 10–24.

Sawyer, A. (2011). Let's talk: a narrative of mental illness, recovery, and the psychotherapist's personal treatment. *Journal of Clinical Psychology: In session*, *67*, 8, 776–88.

Schultz, D. and Flasher, L. (2011). Charles Taylor, Phronesis and medicine: ethics and interpretation in illness narrative. *Journal of Medicine and Philosophy*, *36*, 4, 394–409.

Taylor, C. (2003). Narrating practice: reflective accounts and the textual construction of reality,' *Journal of Advanced* Nursing, 42, 3, 244–51.

Thombre, A., & Rogers, E. M. (2009). Transformative experiences of cancer survivors. In Maggie Wills (Ed.,) *Communicating spirituality in health care*. Cresskill, NJ: Hampton Press.

White, M. (2007). *Maps of narrative practice*. New York: W. W. Norton.

Young, K. G. (1987). *Taleworlds and storyrealms: The phenomenology of narrative*. Boston: Martinus Nijhoff.

Chapter Three

A Decade Navigating Food Allergies

A Mother's Narrative

Courtney Waite Miller

This chapter is a personal narrative of the first ten years of my son's life and his daily battle with food allergies. I hope to encourage compassion for those with food allergies, and promote dialogue (Ellis & Bochner, 2000) by providing an insider account (Adams & Manning, 2015) of the diagnosis and daily management of food allergies from a layperson's perspective (e.g., Carstensen, Papps, & Thompson, 2018; Lauritzen, 2004). I describe Carter's life as the patient and mine as his mother and advocate. I organize the chapter into seven parts, each reflecting a distinct but interrelated period in our lives and his medical care. The story begins with an account of my life while pregnant with him.

    For those not familiar, a food allergy is an adverse reaction to a food that involves the immune system. The most common food allergens are eggs, milk, peanuts, tree nuts, soybeans, wheat, fish, and shellfish. Reactions can range from mild, such as hives or itching, to life threatening, such as anaphylaxis. Anaphylactic allergic reactions often involve hives, swelling, lowered blood pressure and can result in shock when severe. Anaphylactic reactions typically involve more than one body system and can be fatal. These reactions require epinephrine and immediate medical attention. Each year 30,000 Americans require emergency treatment due to food allergies and approximately 150–200 die from allergic reactions to food. A small amount of an allergenic food, such as cross contact from a trace amount of allergenic food during manufacturing, preparation, or serving, can produce a severe allergic reaction (U.S. Food & Drug Administration, 2018). Currently, there is no FDA-approved treatment for food allergy (Tilles & Petroni, 2018). The only treatment is strict avoidance and rescue therapy for exposure, such as injectable epinephrine (Kim, Sinacore, & Pongracic, 2005).

A GOOD PROFESSOR, MOTHER, AND PATIENT

In the winter of 2006 I was twenty-nine years old and in my second year of a tenure-track position at a small liberal arts college in the Midwest. I loved teaching and was publishing some too. My husband and I had been married for two and a half years. He had a job he enjoyed and was earning his MBA at night. All the pieces seemed to be in place. We began to talk about having a baby. We knew we wanted children, but like other academic women (e.g., Acker & Armenti, 2004), I struggled with the "right" time. Is two years on the job too soon to have a baby? Would a baby hurt my chance of earning tenure? Would I regret waiting to have children if we later had trouble conceiving? These were recurring questions for me during this time.

None of these questions mattered by the spring of 2007 when I learned I was pregnant. I went into full research mode, reading everything I could about pregnancy and birth. I signed up for several classes at the hospital and felt prepared for my first appointment with the obstetrician several weeks later. She ran through a list of dos and don'ts. I listened carefully, determined to be a good patient and mother. In the list she mentioned not eating peanuts while pregnant. She said some research had linked that with children later developing allergies to peanuts (Hourihane, Dean, & Warner, 1996). I was surprised by this information. I had not heard or read this anywhere, but I quickly decided I would not eat peanuts while pregnant. Doctor's orders right? Looking back, however, I do not think I thought this warning really applied to me. Food allergies? I did not know much about allergies in general and we did not have any family history of food allergies. But, trying to follow all instructions, I did not eat peanuts for at least six months. I ate a few other nuts on salads or in desserts because my doctor never mentioned anything about those. Toward the end of my pregnancy, I began craving chocolate peanut butter ice cream. I did give in and ate the ice cream.

For several years, I felt guilty about eating this ice cream. I worried I "gave" Carter an allergy to peanuts by not following my doctor's directions. I also ate peanuts while breastfeeding and worried that maybe, again, I could be the cause of his allergy. Now, more recent research has shown that mothers who ate peanuts five times a week or more while pregnant had the *lowest* risk of developing a peanut allergy (Frazier, Camargo Jr., Malspeis, Willett, & Young, 2014). Should I have eaten *more* peanuts? It appears that I should have, but my doctor told me what she thought was best at the time and I complied.

After Carter's diagnosis, I read the initial study that was the basis for my obstetrician's recommendation. The conclusion was tenuous, at best. I wish I had done my own research and asked more questions. At the time, I was disappointed in my doctor as a scientist but more so in myself. I am trained to research and teach students how to critically evaluate journal articles. Why didn't I do that myself?

Objectively, I know the nuts I ate (or did not eat) *alone* did not give Carter food allergies. Research is pointing to a constellation of factors, including genetics (e.g., National Academies of Sciences, Engineering, & Medicine, 2017). Still, a mother's guilt is sometimes hard to overcome (Carstensen, Papps, & Thompson, 2018). I don't know that I will ever fully absolve myself of any responsibility for Carter's allergies.

Carter was born December 21, 2007. My due date was December 20. I remember my husband calling me before leaving work that day and asking if I felt any signs of labor. I told him I was working on a conference paper and to take his time coming home. No one goes into labor on her due date. Wrong! I went into labor several hours later, still writing the conference paper. My co-author often jokes about how I suddenly quit responding to her emails. She knew I had to be in labor because it is so unlike me.

I was in labor almost twenty-four hours and had a difficult birth. I developed a fever and was treated with IV antibiotics. I was upset the two nights I spent in the hospital, feeling I may have failed my son in some way. Instead of being joyful, I cried. At the time, I did not even know that some research has linked antibiotic use to food allergies (Metsala, Lundqvist, Virta, Kaila, Gissler, &Virtanen, 2013, see also Marrs, Bruce, Logan, Rivett, Perkin, Lack, & Flohr, 2013). I just had this nonspecific thought that I did not do a good job. I now feel guilty about that too. If I was better or faster at giving birth, might my son not have food allergies?

SEARCHING FOR ANSWERS

Carter was a content baby. He slept in three or four hour stretches and loved being held. I often wore him in a carrier on my chest, even to work. At the time, my college did not provide paid family leave. My dean was able to (unofficially) give me one course release but that was it. Teaching during my college's January term was optional for me because I met my fall teaching requirements. That meant I had about six weeks off before returning to work. Fortunately, my husband's company provided four weeks of paid leave. With help from my parents we all shared in child care that semester.

I breastfed Carter so when he woke in the night hungry, I got out of bed to feed him. My husband slept soundly through this every time, many times to my frustration! The three- and four-hour stretches of sleep started to get to me after about eight weeks. I remember a foggy haze of just getting by each day and many details from that time are fuzzy. One memory, however, is vivid—recognizing my own fallibility. I had never met my mental or physical limit like this before. There were days I did not teach well, could not recall information I needed, or was just slow in processing information. I made a few mistakes I would not normally make. I remember having the realization that all people, including doctors, must experience this at times when their personal and professional lives collide. Maybe naïve, I had never considered doctors as imperfect, fallible beings before. Now I viewed all people differently, with an empathy I had not had before. This awareness stuck with me. I learned to question doctors and understand that they make mistakes too. Medicine is an art and a science.

As an infant, my son had a series of skin rashes. Three pediatricians in our practice treated his rash with antibiotics and prescribed assorted creams, but none of their interventions worked long term. Frustrated, I found a pediatric dermatologist in the area and begged her office for an appointment. Upon a quick examination of Carter, she said to stop the antibiotics and prescribed a cream that treated his rash and prevented future rashes. That was my first lesson in advocacy and seeking specialists when necessary. I now knew I could not always rely on doctors to have all the right answers.

To this day, we are unsure what caused the rash. I now think the rashes were a reaction to food I ate and passed through to Carter in my breast milk. Or maybe a reaction to food I ate while holding or wearing him, but no one mentioned this possibility at the time. I also feel guilty about the antibiotics he took. I wish I had seen a specialist sooner. I did find a new pediatrician.

My son also developed a persistent cough at nine months of age and chronic ear infections from his first birthday on. His new pediatrician and other doctors in her practice prescribed medicines to treat the cough and ear infections. Nothing worked. Carter continued coughing and had persistent fluid in his ears. He often woke up at night screaming in pain.

Impatient and exhausted, I made an appointment with a pediatric ear, nose, and throat (ENT) doctor my friend suggested. It took several weeks to secure an appointment with him. The day of our appointment he was running an hour behind schedule. When he finally entered the room, he quickly examined Carter and asked me if he attended day care. I said that he did. "Well, get him out of day care!" he responded with frustration and what I perceived to be incriminating eyes. "The next steps will be even stronger antibiotics or an operation to put tubes in his ears."

I fought back tears as I left his office and drove home. In my sleep-deprived, emotional state, his statement felt like a referendum on me working. He could have just as easily meant that we should get a baby sitter instead, but it did not feel like that to me at the time. Was I selfish for wanting to work? Should I consider quitting? I called my mom with tears flowing by this time. She encouraged me to keep working and said she would watch Carter through the winter cold and flu season. Mom to the rescue, even at thirty years old!

As I reflect on this time, I realize I did not call my husband. I perceived child care to be my problem to solve, just as the managerial women Buzzanell, Meisenbach, Remke, Liu, Bowers, and Conn (2005) interviewed. I automatically enacted the good working mother ideology they describe. Without knowing it, I replicated a traditional division of labor and inequitable contributions to child care. Much of this division persists today.

During that time, the infections in Carter's ears cleared, but the fluid did not. The cough improved some. Going the specialist route once again, I took my son to see a pediatric allergist. She thought he might have asthma and gave him a prescription for that. She also tested him for environmental allergies, but the tests were negative. We still did not have answers or a cure.

We took a family vacation to Florida in May right after my semester ended. We enjoyed the beach, pool, and eating out. Looking back, it was the freest and closest to "normal" we would ever be as a family. We flew without concern and spontaneously ate out at several restaurants. We now only fly one airline and eat at a handful of restaurants. Everything is planned and researched. Nothing can be left to chance. We also do not travel internationally or to locations where it might be difficult to buy food or seek medical treatment (see Cummings, Knibb, King, & Lucas, 2010 for a review of the psychosocial impact of food allergy on children and their families). Of course, at the time, I assumed all family vacations would be like this and did not know to appreciate the freedom. I am embarrassed to admit that I am sometimes resentful of the limitations Carter's allergies have put on our lives. I am often sad for the family life I thought we would have.

THE FIRST DIAGNOSIS

When we returned home, Carter had another ear infection and he was given more antibiotics. The two of us were home one afternoon that week and he was asking for a snack. Without really thinking about it, I gave him a mini peanut butter sandwich cracker. It was the size of a nickel, maybe even a dime. He asked for another and I gave it to him. Seconds later, he began profusely vomiting and had a rash on his face. I calmed him, gave him a bath, and cleaned up. By then, he was fine. I called my husband. We wondered if it was the peanut butter that made him sick, or maybe it was the new antibiotics, or a stomach bug? We did not know enough to worry. Or maybe we were in denial.

Looking back with knowledge I now have, we are very lucky nothing worse happened to Carter. He could have died from that reaction. I did not know anything about food allergies then. Food allergies were not a topic of conversation in 2009 as they seem to be now. I feel so stupid and reckless for how I handled that situation. I simply did not know any better. After reading medical research (e.g., Abdurrahman et al., 2013), I know I am not alone in my poor management of his initial reaction.

I did make an appointment with Carter's allergist, to be safe. At the appointment, I explained what happened with the crackers. She said she was almost positive Carter had a peanut allergy. She said she often performs skin prick tests as part of a diagnosis but did not want to do that in his case, given the severity of his initial reaction. She ordered a blood test to confirm the peanut allergy and added tests for allergies to all tree nuts. At the time, I remember not knowing the distinction or maybe just never thinking about it. Tree nuts are nuts that grow on trees (e.g., almonds, walnuts, pecans, pistachios, cashews, etc.) whereas peanuts grow in the ground. She explained that individuals with peanut allergies sometimes have other nut allergies. She gave us a prescription for an Epi-Pen injector and a nurse showed me how to use it. I left her office in a daze.

I drove Carter to a satellite outpatient center affiliated with a children's hospital. The technician asked me to hold him down while she drew blood from his arm. At first, I tried holding him on my lap. He struggled so hard she could not get the needle in correctly. She tried again with me holding him in a bear hug with all my strength. She was successful but suggested bringing someone with me to help next time. My husband worked long hours, so I always went to medical appointments alone. It never occurred to me to ask for help. I had assumed full responsibility for child care and now medical care without a thought. The technician said, "The results will take about a week. The doctor will call you."

I waited a week and did not hear back from the doctor. When I called the office, the receptionist said, "A doctor will have to call you." That is never good news. The doctor called around nine o'clock that night. "Your son has a severe peanut allergy. I've rarely seen levels this high in a child so young. He also tested positive for all tree nuts. Avoid all nuts—a fraction of a peanut could cause a life-threatening reaction. Go to some related websites for more information [she indicated which to go to]. Maybe join a support group for moms of kids with food allergies. He must always have two Epi-Pens with him. Any questions?"

Any questions? I did not even know where to begin. I remember asking some question about labels on packages, but that was it. I was devastated. I immediately went through our pantry cabinet. The first items were obvious discards; peanut butter, gone; trail mix, gone; granola bars, gone. Then I started reading labels on every package. Several items had statements saying they might contain nuts, including dried fruit, multi-grain bread, and a package of cookies. Some items did not have an allergen statement. Did that mean they were safe for Carter to eat? I felt isolated and solely responsible for keeping my child safe and alive, not unlike other parents in my position (Abdurrahman et al., 2013; Allergy New Zealand, 2012).

I went to the websites the doctor suggested and found more information on my own. I learned that up to fifteen million people in the United States have food allergies, and that rates among children are increasing. An estimated one in thirteen children has a food allergy (see www.foodallergy.org for more information). I ordered several books on Amazon and found a local POCHA (Parents of Children Who Have Allergies) group. I learned that food labeling guidelines are voluntary. Food manufacturers can choose to provide information about their manufacturing and packaging processes but are not required to (U.S. Food & Drug Association, 2006). The only way to know if a food is safe for Carter is to call or email each company or find this information on a company website. I spent hours doing this the next morning and discarded more food. Carter played happily, oblivious to his diagnosis. How would I explain this to him? I fought back tears as I read him his favorite book about construction vehicles that afternoon.

The day after Carter's diagnosis, we had two college friends and their families coming to stay with us. I knew from experience that parents travel with food for their kids. I emailed both of my friends telling them about Carter's allergies, asking them not to bring nuts or anything that might have nuts in it. One friend emailed back with a sympathetic message of support and a promise not to bring *any* food into our house. Her support meant a lot to me and I was grateful for the easy cooperation. The other friend responded differently. Her son was about one year old and was on a special diet for digestive issues. She said she could not come to my house if her son could not eat. Could not eat? That was not what I said, but that is what she understood. I said, "I am sure we can make it work so that all the kids can eat," but I was hurt and surprised by her reaction. That was my first taste of disapproval and unwillingness to accommodate Carter's allergies. As is common in the management of health issues, this affected our relationship and other relationships too (e.g., Miller-Day, 2011).

FINDING OUR WAY

Before the diagnosis, we planned for Carter to go back to day care two days a week during the summer of 2009. I needed to get back into my research as my mid-probationary review was looming. I called the home day care provider and explained Carter's allergy. I asked, "Can I send him with his Epi-Pen and food?" She was reassuring and welcoming. She had a background in food service and easily understood the requirements. I felt one hurdle had been crossed and was relieved. Maybe this would not be as difficult as I feared.

That relief did not last. Carter had an ear infection in less than a month. This time the pediatrician said, "I think he needs ear tubes." She referred us to a different pediatric ENT doctor. In contrast to the other ENT doctor, this doctor was kind and empathic. He shared, "I know how stressful a surgery sounds, but placing tubes is a very short operation with almost no recovery time." He explained, "Without the tubes, Carter is just going to keep getting ear infections, especially since this one occurred in the summer outside of the regular cold and flu season." I remember asking the doctor what he would do if Carter were his child. This has become a question I frequently ask of doctors. It seems to cut to the heart of the decision by blending a more objective medical decision with the emotions that often accompany a surgery or treatment. He stated, "I would get the tubes if Carter were my child." That made the decision easier for me.

The doctor's surgery schedule was booked until September 1, the first day of my Tuesday/Thursday classes for that semester. I briefly thought about asking for another appointment, but the ear infections were so painful for Carter. His speech also was starting to show delays, most likely due to the way the fluid on his ears was affecting his hearing. As I look back, the thought of my husband taking him for the surgery, or us taking him together, never crossed my mind. I made the appointment and the necessary adjustments at work. Thankfully my department chair was understanding and supportive and we had the resources to pay for the surgery. I know many others do not.

The operation was as quick as the doctor said it would be. I only spent a few minutes in the family waiting room before the doctor came out to tell me the surgery went well. It was a few more minutes until I could see Carter in recovery. When I saw him, he was a bit confused but soothed by a juice box. I was able to take him home a few hours later. He took his usual nap that afternoon and woke up as if nothing had happened.

I was hoping this was the end of illnesses for Carter and that tubes would be the miracle several friends said they would be. Unfortunately, that was not the case. Carter had several more ear infections. Those could be treated with antibiotic ear drops because the tubes allowed the fluid to drain from his ears. Carter then started developing recurring sinus infections. The infections were probably prevented or treated before by the frequent use of antibiotics. The allergist was worried enough to order tests of his immune system. This time Carter did not fight the blood draw. It was almost as though he knew it was pointless to do so, even at two years of age. Thankfully, his immune function tests were normal. That did not explain the infections.

The ENT doctor suggested another surgery to remove Carter's adenoid. He also said we should repeat the allergy tests Carter had when he was younger. I quickly made an appointment for allergy testing, hoping to avoid another surgery. This was the turning point for us. Carter endured quite a few scratch tests on his skin, followed by intradermal tests in which a small needle with allergens on it is placed under the skin. He tested positive to just about everything indoors and out, including dust, cats, dogs, trees, grass, and weeds. The allergist prescribed a daily antihistamine and a steroid nose spray. She also said, "We have to work to remove allergens from his environment." She gave me pamphlets about how to do this and recommended products to buy.

The allergist asked, "Do you have any pets?" I answered, "no," but then thought about his day care. The day care was on the second-floor apartment of a two-story building. The woman who ran it lived on the first floor with her dog. My son never interacted with the dog. However, the apartment shared vents and stairs. When I told the allergist this, she curtly responded, "He must be removed from day care immediately." She believed this constant irritation to be a major cause of his sinus infections and chronic cough.

We withdrew Carter from day care and once again my mom watched him until we could hire a nanny. Once more, I was grateful we had the resources to do this. We found a nanny and had smooth sailing for several months. I was relieved to have a diagnosis and cause for Carter's symptoms, but also felt tremendous guilt about him going to day care. Going there was a huge component to his near-constant illness. I kept trying to reassure myself that there was no way we could have known this before because he tested negative to these allergens the first time. My husband kept telling me the same thing. However, I had lingering doubts that I somehow could have prevented this if I had listened to the first ENT and removed Carter from day care the year before.

We had an illness-free spring and wonderful summer full of everything a summer should be—the pool, parks, and plenty of downtime. I also became pregnant with our second child. Life felt much easier. We still had to think about the food allergies every day but having Carter healthy was such an improvement. I felt great during the pregnancy and was able to prepare my tenure portfolio while spending lots of time with Carter.

In the fall of 2010, Carter attended a preschool program for two-year olds two mornings a week. I instructed his teacher and her assistant about his allergies. They were accepting and thoughtful. It was a Montessori-based program, so food was a large component of their curriculum. We worked together to make the environment safe for him. I bought new knives and cutting boards for the classroom and researched safe brands of the dozen or so foods that needed to be purchased each week. It was an easy transition. Carter loved the classes and gained some independence.

Because Carter was turning three in December, it was assumed that he would transition to one of the three-year old classrooms in January along with several other students. That all changed when his teacher called me one afternoon in late November. She was awkward at first, asking me, "Do you really want Carter to move up to the three-year old class? Have you and your husband considered other preschools?" I could not figure out the purpose of her call. Then she came right out and said, "Courtney, the teachers in the three-year old rooms do not want Carter. They do not want to make the accommodations necessary for his safety and I could not live with myself if something happened to him. I am telling you it is not a good choice for him."

Wow. Did not want my son? Did not want to accommodate him? I was stunned, sad, mad, fearful for Carter's future, and grateful for his teacher's honesty all at the same time. I later called the director of the school. I told her "Carter will not be returning in January. I would like our tuition deposit back." I continued, "I am horrified that your teachers do not want to accommodate someone with food allergies. Your preschool is behind the times; so many preschools are nut free now." She argued back with me about international food tasting days and other food-related stations integral to their curriculum. Those were worth a risk to a child's life at school? She also insisted, "I cannot control what older, full-day students bring for lunch and I can't refund your deposit. The school has already factored the revenue into our budget." Looking back, I do not know how I managed to stay calm during the call. I am angry even now.

About thirty minutes after I talked with the director, my son's teacher called me again. "The director called upset with me for telling you about the three-year old classrooms. She said I'm going to get the school sued. I did not think you would repeat what I told you." I promised somewhat bitterly, "I am not going to take any legal action against the school. I do not want Carter in that school now anyway." Now I wish I had acted against the school. What they were doing was discriminatory and dangerous. As much as it hurt, I was *lucky* my son's teacher called to tell me how the teachers felt about my son. What about other children without the benefit of a program for two-year old children, or a teacher like ours? I have attempted to make up for my failings here in other situations.

A WAY OF LIFE

Shortly before Christmas in 2010, the president of our college called to tell me he planned to recommend me to the Board of Trustees for tenure. I missed his call because I was downtown at my obstetrician's office, now eight months pregnant. I was thrilled and relieved not to worry about tenure anymore. I also received a call from a preschool at the early childhood center of a university near our home. I put my son's name on their waiting list when he was six months old and they now had a spot for him. It was perfect timing.

The school was nut free, and they could not have been more welcoming to us.

My second son was born in late January 2011, eight days after my due date. This time I had about four weeks off from work. This was a quiet period in Carter's health and allergies—and much needed at that time. We settled into a routine with two kids. The lack of sleep was not such a shock to my system this time around, and I asked for help when I needed it.

We continued regular checkups with Carter's allergist. I had read about a new blood test that measured one's immune response to the individual components of a peanut. There are multiple potentially allergenic components of peanuts, but only a few are related to severe reactions, such as anaphylaxis. One protein, Ara h 2, is especially predictive (e.g., Nicolaou et al., 2010). From what I understood, a patient could have a high IgE level (Immunoglobulin E; an elevated IgE indicates that an allergic process is present to the allergen tested), but not react to peanuts, at least not severely. That is because the high IgE values could be in response to proteins in the peanuts not known to cause severe allergic reactions. This test also would tell us if my son was one of the approximately 20 percent of children likely to outgrow their peanut allergy (Begin, Paradis, Paradis, & Des Roches, 2013).

When I told people, "My son has a peanut allergy," just about everyone asked, "Will he outgrow it?" Often they shared "I think he will" or "I know someone who outgrew a food allergy." It became annoying to me over time and I struggled to be polite. I knew the chance of my son outgrowing his allergy was very small, due to his high IgE level to peanuts and the overall low rate of children outgrowing peanut allergies. However, when I read about this test, I somehow lifted my hopes up that a) he could be among the lucky 20 percent or b) he was only allergic to the harmless proteins in a peanut and not the ones that cause severe reactions. My doctor agreed to order the test. We left with a kit and a phone number for a nurse to come to our house and draw Carter's blood. The blood was then FedExed to a lab in Michigan. The test was $300, and insurance did not cover it.

We decided to do the test right before Carter's fifth birthday, reasoning that some kids outgrow the allergy by this age (e.g., Begin et al., 2013). The results also would provide useful information to have before Carter started kindergarten the following year. Once again, we were told the results would take about a week. When more than a week went by, I called the office. One of our doctor's fellows called me back. I hoped he was the bearer of good news and really thought he might be. That is until he said, "These are exactly the results you don't want. Not only has your son's IgE level increased by five times, he is extremely reactive to the protein most associated with anaphylactic reactions. Ironically, the only protein he is not allergic to is one that does not seem to have much effect on one's allergic response."

My hopes were dashed in less than sixty seconds. In the week we waited for the test, I started to fantasize about going to bakeries, ice cream shops, and birthday parties where Carter could eat the cake. I thought maybe we could spontaneously go to a restaurant. The doctor made it sound like the chance of that ever happening was close to zero. I was beside myself. I do not know why I let myself become hopeful. My husband said he expected those results. To him, the test was what he already knew. I wish I had known to be more pessimistic. I think I did not want to believe this allergy was a lifelong sentence for Carter.

PUBLIC SCHOOL

Before we knew it, it was time for Carter to start kindergarten at a public school. We had grown comfortable with his nut-free preschool and I was nervous for this transition. The school nurse called me about two weeks before school started. We went over Carter's allergies and the school's typical allergy protocol, which was not much. Every item seemed up for negotiation and debate. My PhD in communication and undergraduate training in argumentation was quite helpful during this call! By the end, we agreed that he would not sit at a peanut-free table, isolated from other students. The nurse admitted that no one sat there. We worked out a plan for him to sit on an aisle with a placemat for his food and not near other kids eating nuts. We also agreed that his teacher would not let other kids eat nuts in the classroom and that kids would wipe or wash their hands after lunch. I wondered why there was not a more formal protocol for this process. Why was each item a debate? I worried about other kids whose parents did not have the knowledge or wherewithal to advocate as I did. I looked up other school districts and found that they had specific allergy protocols in place. Why didn't our district have one?

Around this same time, I had met a mom whose two children also had nut allergies. She happened to be a writer and had similar experiences negotiating with another school in our district. She was a friend to two other mothers of kids with food allergies, one an attorney and the other a psychologist. Together, they learned that our school district was in violation of state law. All schools were required to have a food allergy management protocol in place. Those three moms led the effort to develop a food allergy protocol for our school district. I was able to help with an early draft. By the next school year, the food allergy protocol was in place. It mostly put an end to the individual negotiations on accommodations. All I had to do was refer others, including the school principal, to the policy and the necessary accommodations were made, albeit begrudgingly in some cases. I was grateful, relieved, and in awe of these moms.

What the policy limited, but did not end, was food for classroom celebrations. Sadly, these hour-long parties were not safe for kids with food allergies. There was little control of what food was served, and how it was served. Children also did not wash their hands before eating. Hand washing is a must for individuals with food allergies. When my son was in kindergarten, I signed up to bring the food for every party and attended the parties to serve the food myself. I made sure my son cleaned his hands. Due to a separate wellness policy, the food choices were limited to "healthy" options such as cheese, crackers, and fruit. Many of the kids did not eat the food provided. They either did not like it or were not hungry. It was a waste of resources and an unnecessary risk for kids with food allergies. I informed the nurse and principal of this, but nothing changed.

In first grade, my son's teacher decided to make her classroom food free for all celebrations. In addition to my son, she had three other kids with food allergies in her class. She said the food was not worth the risk. This was such a weight off my shoulders, but only helped her students. Food allergy kids in other classrooms were still served food at parties. This did not seem right and I set about changing it. It took a lot of talking and my training in persuasive communication again, but the principal finally agreed not to serve food at parties, except for popsicles at field day. I couldn't win that one! Food allergy kids instantly became safer at school. Ironically, three years later, it is now a district-wide goal to have all in-school events food free within three years. The multi-year plan is necessary to phase in this requirement because food is so ingrained in many school cultures. Frustratingly slow, but still progress.

TURNING THE TIDE

In my research on food allergies, I read about an experimental treatment called Oral Immunotherapy (OIT). OIT works by slowly desensitizing one's body to an allergen through eating the allergen in controlled amounts, starting from microscopic parts and building to whole servings of a food (for more information, see www.oit101.org). The treatment takes place in an allergist's office or as part of a clinical trial. OIT is still new and using it in private practice is somewhat controversial. Currently, there are only two allergists in the state of Illinois offering this treatment. OIT is in clinical trials at several hospitals but is not recognized as a food allergy treatment by the FDA. None of this was enough to stop me after reading the OIT success stories in academic journals and online.

I made consultation appointments with both doctors in Illinois. We are fortunate to be able to drive to two OIT allergists in about an hour and have comprehensive health insurance. Many patients fly or drive long distances to doctors for this treatment, which takes a minimum of twenty-five office visits to complete, and not all insurance companies cover it. Both doctors have long waiting lists and are selective about the patients they accept. They must be sure all instructions will be followed, and that all parties are committed to the treatment. It is too dangerous otherwise. Both doctors agreed to put Carter on their waiting lists. I think being a professor really helped his odds of receiving treatment, especially when I started referring to specific studies from medical journals! One of the doctors was particularly excited about OIT research and traveled around the country to meet other OIT providers and learn from their experiences. His enthusiasm for the benefits of OIT and confidence in his ability to treat Carter was remarkable. Carter trusted him and his nurse immediately.

Carter began OIT with this doctor in the fall of 2016. The treatment starts with a full day of twenty "doses" of peanut protein mixed in grape Kool-Aid. Each dose increases the amount of peanut consumed. The treatment works by desensitizing one's immune system without it realizing what is occurring and reacting. Carter was calm and brave throughout the day. I was nervous, but so ready for the miracle many families said OIT provided (e.g., Arasi et al., 2014; Otani et al., 2014). We left with a "dose" for Carter to take at home twice a day for a week. This dose had a fraction of a peanut in it. We returned to the allergist's office every week for the dose to be increased under the doctor's supervision. The Kool-Aid solution is the first phase of the treatment, followed by peanut flour, and then actual peanuts. After a dose is eaten, the patient must be directly observed for an hour and cannot increase their heart rate or body temperature for two hours. This "rest period" is extremely important. The doses also had to be spaced no less than nine hours apart and no more than fifteen hours apart. It took a lot of planning and some early mornings to make these requirements work. My husband came to one of the treatment appointments and took an active role in following the protocol at home. The demands of the treatment helped my husband share in Carter's medical care. I could not do it alone.

It was surreal to buy peanuts for this treatment. I had come to hate peanuts. I still do. Such a tiny, silly thing had caused Carter so much trouble and threatened his life. Carter "graduated" from peanut OIT in the spring of 2017 and now must eat peanuts every day for the foreseeable future to maintain his immunity. I am still in disbelief some days. We also found he is not allergic to some of the tree nuts his blood and skin test positive for such as almonds, Brazil nuts, and macadamia nuts. He is allergic to pecans, walnuts, cashews, and pistachios. He is likely allergic to sesame seeds and sunflower seeds too, so we still must be careful where and what he eats. But our worlds have opened a bit and we are less fearful. We no longer panic at the sight of a peanut. We have added some new foods, restaurants, and experiences that would not have been possible without OIT. OIT is available for other allergens, such as tree nuts, milk, and sesame seeds.

Eating peanuts every day is a tremendous chore for Carter. He absolutely hates how peanuts taste and smell. As his doctor says, "the primitive, reptile part of his brain knows to avoid peanuts" and we must work against that protective instinct every day. That sacrifice is worth it to Carter for the safety and freedom he has gained. He is now not so worried at school and is thinking about whether he would like to go to a Major League baseball game. In the past, when his T-ball team went to a Sox game and paraded around the field together, we could not consider going. It was way too dangerous but it was hard not to be a part of this event. Now it's safe, but he's not sure he can stand the smell of the peanuts. At least he now he has a choice.

Currently, Carter does not want to do OIT for his other allergies. He does not want to eat more nuts every day and his stomach has become quite sensitive. I sometimes wish he wanted to do more OIT, but my instincts tell me not to push him. I am trying to be patient. We know the treatment option is there, along with several other possible treatments currently in clinical trials. Although the future of his other food allergies is unknown, I am hopeful. I am grateful we could afford the financial burden food allergies cause (Gupta, Holdford, Bilaver, Dyer, Holl, & Meltzer, 2013) and that my education benefitted Carter and our ability to secure treatment for him. I recognize the privilege we have in managing and treating his food allergies.

Our lives have been forever changed by his allergies. I have learned the power of doing my own research, seeking second opinions, and advocating for Carter as a patient. I have seen the benefits of advocating for one child and how that can help many more. He is wise beyond his ten years and thinks more deeply than most. He knows he must make informed decisions about his food allergies every day, and he does. He says he is going to be an allergist when he grows up and is going to offer a *range* of treatments for food allergies. I truly hope his vision is possible for him and the millions of others with food allergies.

REFERENCES

Aburrahman, Z. B., Kastner, M., Wurman, C., Harada, L., Bantock, L., Cruickshank, H., & Waserman, S. (2013). Experiencing a first food allergic reaction: A survey of parent and caregiver perspectives. *Allergy, Asthma & Clinical Immunology, 7*(2), A6. doi:10.1186/1710-1492-9-18.

Acker, S., & Armenti, C. (2004). Sleepless in academia. *Gender & Education, 16*(1), 3–24. doi:10.1080/0954025032000170309.

Adams, T. E., & Manning, J. (2015). Autoethnography and family research. *Journal of Family Theory & Review, 7*(4), 350–66. doi:10.1111/jftr.12116.

Allergy New Zealand, (2012). 2012 report. What is the prevalence of food allergy in New Zealand? Retrieved from http://www.allergy.org.nz/site/allergynz/What%20is%20the%20 prevalence%20of%20food%20allergy%20in%20New%20Zealand.pdf.

Arasi, S., Otani, I. M., Klingbeil, E., Begin, P., Kearney, C., Dominguez, T. L. R. . . . Nadeau, K. C. (2014). Two year effects of food allergen immunotherapy on quality of life in caregivers of child with food allergies. *Allergy, Asthma & Clinical Immunology, 10*(1), 1–16. doi:10.1186/1710-1492-10-57.

Begin, P., Paradis, L., Paradis, J., & Des Roches, A. (2013). Natural resolution of peanut allergy: A 12-year longitudinal follow-up study. *Journal of Allergy and Clinical Immunology: In Practice, 1*(5), 528–30. doi:10.1016/j.jaip.2013.05.008.

Buzzanell, P. M., Meisenbach, R., Remke, R., Liu, M., Bowers, V., & Conn, C. (2005). The good working mother: Managerial women's sensemaking and feelings about work–family issues. *Communication Studies, 56*, 261–85. doi:10.1080/105109705001.81389

Carstensen, C., Papps, E., & Thompson, S. (2018). When a child is diagnosed with severe allergies: An autoethographic account. *Nursing Practice in New Zealand, 34*(2), 6–16.

Cummings, A. J., Knibb, R. C., King, R. M., & Lucas, J. S. (2010). The psychosocial impact of food allergy and food hypersensitivity in children, adolescents and their families: A review. *Allergy, 65* (8), 933–45. doi:10.1111/j.1398-9995.2010.02342.x.

Ellis, C., & Bochner, A. P. (2000). Autoethnography, personal narrative, reflexivity: Researcher as subject. In N. K. Denzin & Y. S. Lincoln (Eds.), *Handbook of Qualitative Research* (2nd Ed.) (pp. 733–68). Thousand Oaks, CA: Sage.

Frazier, A. L., Camargo Jr., C. A., Malspeis, S., Willett, W.C., & Young, M.C. (2014). Prospective study of peripregnancy consumption of peanuts or tree nuts by mothers and the risk of peanut or tree nut allergy in their offspring. *JAMA Pediatrics, 168*(2), 156–62. doi:10.1001/jamapediatrics.2013.4139.

Gupta R., Holdford, D., Bilaver, L., Dyer, A., Holl, J. L., & Meltzer, D. (2013). The economic impact of childhood food allergy in the United States. *JAMA Pediatrics, 167* (11), 1026–31. doi:10.1001/jamapediatrics.2013.2376.

Hourihane, J., Dean, T., & Warner, J. (1996). Peanut allergy in relation to heredity, maternal diet, and other atopic diseases: Results of a questionnaire survey, skin prick testing, and food challenges. *BMJ: British Medical Journal, 313* (7056), 518–21. doi:10.1136/bmj.313.7056.518.

Kim, J. S, Sinacore, J. M., & Pongracic, J. A. (2005). Parental use of Epi-pen for children with food allergies. *Journal of Allergy and Clinical Immunology, 116* (1), 164–69. doi:10.1016/j.jaci.2005.03.039.

Lauritzen, S. (2004). Lay voices on allergic conditions in children: Parent's narratives and negotiation of a diagnosis. *Social Science & Medicine, 58* (7), 1299–308. doi:10.1016/j.jaci.2005.03.039.

Marrs, T., Bruce, K. D., Logan, K., Rivett, D. W., Perkin, M. R., Lack, G., & Flohr, C. (2013). Is there an association between microbial exposure and food allergy? A systematic review. *Pediatric Allergy and Immunology, 24* (4). 311–20. doi:10.1111/pai.12064.

Metsala, J., Lundqvist, A., Virta, L. J., Kaila, M., Gissler, M., & Virtanen, S. M. (2013). Mother's and offspring's use of antibiotics and infant allergy to cow's milk. *Epidemiology, 24* (2), 303–9. doi:10.1097/EDE.0b013e31827f520f.

Miller-Day, M. (2011). *Family communication, connections, and health transitions: Going through this together.* New York and Bern, Switzerland: Peter Lang.

National Academies of Sciences, Engineering, and Medicine. (2017). *Finding a path to safety in food allergy: Assessment of the global burden, causes, prevention, management, and public policy.* Washington, DC: The National Academies Press. doi:10.17226/23658.

Nicolaou, N., Poorafshar, M., Murray, C., Simpson, A., Winell, H., Kerry, G., . . . Custovic, A. (2010). Allergy or tolerance in children sensitized to peanut: P revalence and differentiation using component-resolved diagnostics. *Journal of Allergy and Clinical Immunology, 125* (1), 191–97. doi:10.1016/j.jaci.2009.10.008.

Otani, I. M., Bégin, P., Kearney, C., Dominguez, T. L., Mehrotra, A., Bacal, L. R., Wilson, S., ... Nadeau, K. (2014). Multiple-allergen oral immunotherapy improves quality of life in caregivers of food-allergic pediatric subjects. *Allergy, Asthma, and Clinical Immunology, 10* (1), 25. doi:10.1186/1710-1492-10-25.

Tilles, S. A., & Petroni, D. (2018). FDA-approved peanut allergy treatment: The first wave is about to crest. *Annals of Allergy, Asthma & Immunology, 121* (2), 145–49. doi:10.1016/j.anai.2018.06.005.

U.S. Food and Drug Administration (2006, July 18). *Food allergen labeling and Consumer Protection Act of 2004 questions and answers*. Retrieved from https://www.fda.gov/Food/GuidanceRegulation/ucm106890.htm#q13.

U.S. Food and Drug Administration (2018, September 26). *Food allergens: what you need to know*. Retrieved from https://www.fda.gov/Food/IngredientsPackagingLabeling/FoodAllergens/ucm079311.htm.

Chapter Four

Growing Up with a Chronic Illness

Easily Concealed, Even Easier to Forget

Kasey Bruss and Jennifer Morey Hawkins

This health narrative invites readers on a journey that starts really at where all my (Bruss) memories begin.[1] I was diagnosed with a childhood kidney cancer at age three and have lived with one kidney and kidney disease in said kidney since then. Having cancer, and going through the surgeries, chemotherapy, and radiation treatments at age three to beat the cancer have had less of an impact than the repercussions of kidney disease and survivor's guilt. Because much happened when I was so young, there are moments I remember vividly and some that I could not give you the slightest detail about. Therefore, some of the moments at the beginning of my story come from memories reconstructed through conversations with my mom.[2] Filling in the blanks where my young mind did not form lasting impressions by talking to my mom doesn't make what happened to me any less real today. Rather, reconstructing the memories provide the opportunity to make sense of how I currently interpret the experiences (McCreight, 2004). As Riessman writes, "The truths of narrative accounts lie not in their faithful representation of a past world, but in the shifting connections they forge among past, present, and future" (2003, p. 341).

According to a lifespan communication perspective, behavior and understanding change over time (Fisher & Roccotagliata, 2017). Development does not necessarily follow a linear path. Rather, growth occurs in a variety of ways and directions (Baltes, Reese, & Nesselroade, 1988). Through the years of learning more about the early stages of my life, and what I went through, my process of understanding, accepting, and communicating about my experience is far from linear. As "narrators create plots from disordered experience" (Riessman, 1993, p. 4), so I organize this chapter around a chronologically linear plot that connects to my broader and ongoing life story.

When I was younger, I would shy away from telling anyone about my illness. I never told anyone about having one kidney. I kept it hidden. Looking back now, I realize that at the time I didn't want to accept that I was different from everyone else. I didn't want to accept that we were not the same. According to Schmidt, Peterson, and Bullinger (2002), children and adolescents living with chronic disease tend to use technical coping strategies, such as escape-denial. Keeping quiet served me well. As long as I did not talk about my health issues, they did not take the limelight. Back then, and now, concern that the items disclosed might be too much for the other person to handle impacts whether or not I choose to share (Derlega, Winstead, & Folk-Barron, 2000). It's hard to bring having cancer into a conversation because really, when is it ever a "good time" to bring it up? Everyone I tell feels sorry for me. That's not what I'm looking for. I don't want sympathy—I simply want people to know more about me and more about why I am the way that I am.

"Good narratives can be beneficial in making our complex experiences more simple and understandable" (Pennebaker & Seagal 1999, p. 1251). Storytelling helps the storyteller "develop personal resilience" while encouraging the audience to "celebrate the hardiness of research participants" (East, Jackson, O'Brien, & Peters, 2010, p. 20). As I got older, and through the process of writing my story, I have been able to connect the dots more as to how my struggles and triumphs have made me into the resilient person that I am now. I have become more open, and communicate more freely about my past. However, at this point in time I only share my story when people ask, rather than proactively telling it. While I open up more than I have before, I still choose to limit or expand upon the depth of disclosure depending on the person. For example, when I am hanging out with people in the summer in a bikini, people will notice my scar and ask questions. I give them the gist of it saying, "Oh I had cancer when I was little so I had my kidney removed." Really, that's about it. People know the basics. I rarely open up with every struggle I have faced post-cancer treatments. I don't want people to think I want pity or think of me as "damaged."

Putting my life story to paper has empowered me to begin to own my narrative (Harter, Japp, & Beck, 2005) of long-term cancer survivorship. According to Ellingson, not much attention is given to stories from those of us living post cancer, "beyond the initial transition from acute treatment to survivorship" (2017, p. 322). The dominant narrative regarding those diagnosed with cancer is that either their stories end with "happily ever after (cure) or tragically (death), but nothing in between" (Ellingson & Borofka, 2018, p. 8). My story does not end "happily ever after" due to being cancer free. Nor, thankfully, did it end abruptly in death. This personal narrative of life with ongoing health issues after cancer provides a lifespan perspective. I accept everything that has happened to me in my past, acknowledge where I'm at now, and know that I do have a bright future ahead of me, even if I have major gains and losses along the way.

THE START OF IT ALL

This is normal. I was diagnosed at age three with Wilms' tumor, a childhood kidney cancer that affects one in every ten thousand children in the United States (www.stjude.org). This is where memories of my life start. I have no memories before Wilms' tumor. There really is no rhyme or reason as to why or how this kidney cancer developed. The cancer just seems to randomly develop from immature kidney cells. All I've ever known is a life with one kidney, a life with kidney disease, a life as a cancer survivor.

My cancer journey all began when I was entering preschool. To start, I needed to be up-to-date with shots and have a physical. July 8, 1999: My appointment came sooner than originally planned, due to a cancellation. During my appointment, the doctor pushed down on my stomach, a normal routine during a well child exam. Right away, he noticed something was wrong, but he tried to play it off as something not as serious as it ended up being. "Something feels different, I believe it might be her spleen," he stated to my mom. "Just schedule an ultrasound within the next few days and we'll go from there." So, Mom scheduled my ultrasound for the next day, July 9.

I remember lying on an exam table, ice-cold jelly all over my stomach, and an ultrasound tech with tears in her eyes. Looking back, I'm certain those tears were waiting to sneak out and flow. However, the tech was unable to say what she saw—a tumor growing on my left kidney . . . so the tears remained in the wings. At this point, everyone knew something was wrong. The doctor and nurse came into the room, both crying. Through tears, he told my mom, "A tumor is growing on Kasey's kidney.... We are pretty sure it is cancerous." My mom told me she remembers that moment as if it was yesterday. She remembers exactly what she was wearing and how strong my grandma acted around her to try and make her feel better. "I already called, they're waiting for you on the eighth floor at Children's in Minneapolis. Go home, pack a bag and they'll be ready for you when you get there." My mom went home, packed a bag, and called my grandpa to drive the two of us down to the city because she was crying too hard to be able to drive. My grandma took care of my sister and called my dad's parents to let them know what was happening.

The next day, I had emergency surgery. It was a Saturday. Only my family and one other family were in the waiting room. The doctor matter-of-factly told my parents, "The surgery should take about two to three hours."

My mother recently shared with me, "When the surgeon came out forty-five minutes later, there wasn't one doubt in my mind that you had died." The surgeon provided an update, "We were able to see more clearly the extent of the tumor soon after we began. Unfortunately, the tumor has aggressively spread. We were unable to remove the tumor. So, we need to change the treatment plan. Kasey needs to undergo chemo for eight weeks and then we'll try surgery again."

Luckily for me, this type of cancer was not life threatening. According to St. Jude's Children's Research Hospital, the long-term survival rate is 85–90 percent, so my odds were looking pretty good, I would say (www.stjude.org). The goal was to get through this little hiccup and get back to being a healthy, happy kiddo. As healthy as I could be, I suppose. After I had my left kidney removed, I completed my six months of chemo and two weeks of radiation. They had to take my entire kidney though, which is not usually what happens with Wilms' tumor. The cancer spread so aggressively throughout my kidney, full removal was the only option. Chemotherapy turned me into a different person. As much as my mom tried to make me eat, food came right back up every time. My hair fell out in chunks until I had nothing left but some stragglers trying their best to make me look "normal"; or at least like a girl, so I didn't have to wear dresses every day to stop people from wondering if I was a boy or a girl. . . . Looking back at pictures now, I don't know why my parents did not just shave my head. I looked like a mess: a barely-alive-type-of-skinny, bald mess.

There are few things that I distinctly remember while all of this was happening. The moments that I do remember, I don't think I will ever be able to forget. I remember the anesthesiologist putting the "gas mask" on me, coated in Dr. Pepper ChapStick. I remember wanting to stay awake because I wanted to watch this crazy organ be pulled out of my body. The anesthesiologist started counting down from ten with me. I didn't even make it to "eight" before I was knocked out. I remember waking up from surgery after having my kidney removed, seeing my mom, and then just falling back asleep. I remember family visiting me. I recall playing cards with my sister; sitting on the edge of my bed looking up to my mother and begging, "Mom, will you bring me ribs and root beer tomorrow when you come?" I honestly couldn't tell you what my obsession with ribs and root beer stemmed from . . . maybe because it reminded me of home? My dad makes the best ribs. Well, he makes the best everything. Ribs drenched in barbeque sauce made me happy. Those ribs made me forget that I was sick and living in a hospital, I guess. I can't eat ribs as often anymore—probably because I overdid it during my stay in the hospital. Barq's root beer, however, is still my jam. It was such a treat to have ribs and root beer during that time when I was eating hospital food for every meal and my only liquids consisted of water and medicine. And, what three-year-old old doesn't love sugar? I also have this very distinct memory of a nurse trying to give me a liquid form of medication and asking, "Do you want orange or grape flavor this time?" "Orange," I answered. I still remember that taste. I can taste it when I am eating an overly sugared orange candy. Without even thinking about it, that orange flavor instantly takes me back into that hospital room. That same hospital room where I jumped out of my bed, IV cart in hand, and stood in front of the bathroom mirror to see a clear bandage across my newly stitched up scar. Looking down, I saw the watery-blood pooling up at the bottom of that bandage. That scar—that surgery—hurt. I remember begging my mom not to make me sit up in my bed. Even when assisted by a bed that could raise my upper body via remote control, sitting up hurt. Maybe that is why I have such a high pain tolerance now? At age three I felt the worst pain I could ever imagine. Still, nothing compares to that pain.

Growing up, I never felt different. Hanging out in that hospital room, day in and day out, getting needles shoved in my arms, having chemo pushed into the port above my heart, puking my guts out from every dose, felt normal. In my little three-year-old mind, I thought this is what every kid did at my age. For a while there, I think it was harder on my parents than it was on me. Therefore, I feel like I should not be proud of being a cancer survivor. I really didn't do anything. I did not feel like I had to fight. I didn't even know that there was the possibility that age three was going to be the longest I lived. Once my kidney was removed and the chemo and radiation were complete, I was back at school doing what other wild preschoolers do; making my parents want to rip their hair out because I did whatever I wanted, whenever I wanted.

THE IN-BETWEEN AND THE ONSET OF SURVIVOR'S GUILT

Growing up, really, the only thing that having cancer stopped me from doing was playing contact sports. Therefore, at age five, I found myself through a different sport when I was cleared to participate in gymnastics. Thank God, because I loved being able to flip around on the floor, swing on the bars, and run around, getting all of my built-up energy out. Eventually, I stopped caring that I couldn't participate in anything else. Gymnastics was what I loved. To be good, I had to be completely dedicated. I didn't have time for anything else.

I had some strange identity crisis when I completed my senior season in gymnastics. I think I was just lost about who I was and who I wanted to be, because I never really was a part of anything else. If I was not a gymnast anymore, who was I? I didn't like identifying myself as a cancer survivor because there are so many people who had it so much worse than I could even imagine. I didn't even know the seriousness of my condition half of the time. I was too young to know that my experiences were not like what all the kids my age were doing. Yes, I felt sick. I just didn't comprehend that my condition was bad.

I do have this weird survivor's guilt. Only recently have I learned that survivor's guilt *is* real. According to Hutson, Hall, and Pack, survivor's guilt is "a valid form of suffering" and is even associated with post-traumatic stress disorder and depression (2015, p. 20). Looking back, I am realizing that I felt guilty when others died.

About a year and a half ago, a girl I grew up with passed away from sarcoma. Megan was eighteen and about to graduate from high school when cancer took her life away. She was adored by so many: with her spunky attitude and vibrant smile. So why didn't she survive? She had already beaten sarcoma once. However, sarcoma decided it was not done with her yet. When people say that cancer is a battle (Frank, 1995), she made that statement look true. Megan would try her hardest to live the life she wanted to, all while going through treatments; trying to act like cancer did not affect her as much as people thought it did. She wanted to come off as strong. She already was. She didn't even need to try. I don't know if I will ever know anyone who will fight harder to stay alive than she did. She rarely went to school her senior year because they were constantly upping her dosage of chemo to try to kill the cancer cells that were viciously taking over her body. In two weeks, the cancer that had started in the left side of her lung had spread. It spread throughout her chest and into her lymph nodes, but she continued to fight on. Megan hated having cancer. She would tell us how much she hated being referred to as "the girl with cancer." She hated how everyone wore the color yellow in honor of her because it represented childhood cancer. She absolutely hated yellow because cancer did not define her. She wanted so much more for her life, but it was taken away from her. She was so excited to go to college and to one day start a family. But toward the end the chemo took its toll. The doctors allowed her to do her chemo treatments in-home when the new school year came around. She felt sicker, weaker, and more irritable than ever before. For a short while prior to her rapid decline, Megan was feeling better. She had shared with me that she started to feel like her old self instead of being so sick and tired all the time anymore. Megan knew the chemo wasn't working. That made her outlook on the treatments even worse. I remember reading Megan's Caringbridge post, written by her mom, stating that her family was absolutely heartbroken that Megan decided she had had enough of the cancer treatments. She was done. Done with chemo, done with radiation, done with trying to kill whatever was taking over her body. She made the decision around Thanksgiving and passed away by the end of December. Her funeral was packed. I think my dad and I went through two Kleenex packages alone in an attempt to slow the constant flow of tears. I can't help but wonder if people question why Megan was taken at age eighteen with so much potential, yet I survived at age three with nothing to my name. I was diagnosed with and survived cancer at such a young age that I didn't fully comprehend the battle. As a survivor, I wonder why I was given an easy way out. Having cancer was not a traumatizing experience for me like it is for so many others who go through it later in life. I didn't understand what I could lose. I don't recall a life before diagnosis.

I feel survivor's guilt more often than I would like to admit. I struggle knowing that I survived, but there are millions of others who did not even have a chance. I struggle to understand how I, once a little weakling three-year-old whose biggest accomplishment at the time of diagnosis and successful surgery was being potty trained, survived this disease at such a young age. Yet, some individuals who are far more accomplished than I could ever dream of did not and do not make it. I question why I survived more than being proud of the fact that I actually did survive. Because I mess up on a daily basis, I can't help but think maybe I have not lived up to the title "cancer survivor?" Like . . . why did I survive?

I don't know why some survive and others do not. Cancer is a sick game of Russian roulette. You just really never know your fate. I always hoped that one day I would have this epiphany and be like, "*This*—this exact reason—is why everything that has happened to me, happened. So, I could do/see/be a part of *this*." But, really, I don't think there is any rhyme or reason behind why people are handed the illnesses they receive. I may have survived cancer once, but there is always the possibility that it will come back; or that the repercussions of having cancer take me. I tell myself all the time that the only thing we are ever fully guaranteed in this life is that we are going to die. That's it. It's dramatic and maybe even a little gloomy, but it's true. And, I'm a realist more than anything else. I try to live like it could happen tomorrow. I just want to have fun while I can and do the things I love. However, I do struggle with the true meaning of "having fun."

THE COLLEGE YEARS

In college, having fun means getting plastered on a Thursday night when The Pub has drinks for 50 cents. The dance floor is the only thing I care about for the night. I live for girl's nights: getting down to some old Shania Twain with my favorite friends. Picture me, several drinks in, with one kidney that has kidney disease: in that moment, not even remembering that that statement is a true fact.

I know drinking isn't good for me when I have kidney disease. I'm basically in escape-denial (Schmidt, Peterson, & Bullinger, 2002) every

Thursday–Sunday, maybe even Wednesday's for those karaoke and $1 shot nights that I just can't say "no" to. I'm in denial about the fact that it is less dangerous for my friends to binge drink than it is for me. I don't want to admit that some nights I should say no to participating in serious shenanigans. I don't want to admit that I do have a chronic disease that should keep me from such shenanigans. It's not the alcohol itself. It's the dehydration caused by drinking alcohol instead of drinking water like a fish.

So many days I forget that I'm missing a kidney because it is honestly all I have ever known. Kidney disease is one of those hidden illnesses. No one would ever know about my condition unless I tell them. I don't tell people often enough for it to constantly be on my mind. I still don't see myself as different, which is why my kidney disease causes problems sometimes. I have yet to damage my kidney to the point of no return. However, I know that keeping up my current habits has the potential of getting me there. It sounds absolutely nuts when I write it down on paper that I really don't pay attention to my kidney disease, but I don't. I don't want to say I am neglecting my health, but I do not know enough about my body to ensure that I am doing everything possible to keep my kidney functioning at its highest potential.

The last I checked, I'm doing as well as I should be. My kidney is doing its job keeping up the good work. I try to compensate for the alcohol consumption by drinking my weight in ounces of water per day, but I don't know if I necessarily get take-backs when it comes to my health. It's honestly kind of stupid of me to act like I'm a responsible human being when I can't even take care of myself properly some days.

INTO THE UNKNOWN

Easily Forgotten

It's interesting to think about the repercussions of cancer treatments. No young child thinks about the long-term effects. At least I know I never did. I wonder if other kids, or family members for that matter, do? According to Wo and Viswanathan "women treated with abdomino-pelvic radiation have an increased rate of uterine dysfunction leading to miscarriage, preterm labor, low birth weight, and placental abnormalities" (2009, p. 1304). Who thinks that far ahead when you are trying to survive right now? Those of us who are in treatment live more in the moment wanting to just beat whatever is trying to take us: but, what if that treatment ruins our future? What if treatments interfere with what we hope our future would hold?

According to the American Cancer Society, when radiation is performed all over the abdomen it can affect ovaries and the uterus (www.cancer.org). My uterus just might not stretch during pregnancy like it should, which increases my risk of miscarriage, low birth-weight babies, and premature births. According to Green et al. (2009), ovarian failure and premature menopause may occur as after-effects of radiation in pediatric cancer patients. Honestly, the thought of being infertile or losing a baby during a pregnancy absolutely terrifies me. My doctor basically told me *if* my body can handle me carrying a baby to full-term, I better get 'er done before twenty-eight. It was not a serious conversation. I remember her telling me, "If it's something you're thinking about, you should probably think about it sooner rather than later . . . I'd say twenty-eight would be your cut off before any pregnancies would become even more high-risk." If I am doing my math correctly, that gives me about six and a half years to find the man of my dreams and pop out a couple of kiddos.

Not only does it scare me to have this timeline, it scares me that someone else, hopefully some guy that I am madly in love with, would go through a pregnancy loss with me without being responsible for the cause. I have a lot of anxiety about this part of my future. I have wanted to be a mom for so long. I have always wanted to be a mom and raise children with a man I love. Because I have this underlying fear and thought in my mind that I must try to have kids as soon as possible, I think I ruin relationships. I find myself rushing in too quickly, getting more serious with someone sooner rather than later. I'm afraid of waiting for later. Honestly, I'm terrified that I'm not following the timeline given to me. The terror hasn't done one good thing for me. I feel bad. I have ruined perfectly fine relationships because of this underlying fear of not falling in love at the right time, waiting too long, or not ultimately having what I have always wanted—a happy marriage with kiddos.

I do not like to make plans because I have learned that they don't work out. However, I would like to have the *option* of having a family later in life. At this point, I really don't know if I want one. I would like to keep my options open in case some dark haired, handsome man decides to sweep me off my feet within the next few years. So far, no one is lining up at my door. Oh and yeah, screaming kids at Target make me want to rip my hair out. Do you see my problem? My favorite thing to do with my problems is pretend I don't have any. I casually sprint as far away as possible.

Thinking about the future scares me. I know that what I do now determines my future. I may only be in stage two kidney disease now, but that is now, not later. Are the nights out with my girlfriends really affecting my kidney that much? Do I *really* have to take my medication every day? I think I can get away with my actions because I've been in the same stage of kidney disease since I was four. Honestly, I don't know how much my logic lines up with actual reality.

I know I do things that I shouldn't be doing. Maybe I *should* care more about my health status. Having to remember to take some medication every single day is hard sometimes; especially when I feel it's really not that important. They took me off medication for three whole months when I was eight. I *know* I need to care more, but with having chronic kidney disease for basically my entire life, it's hard to know any different or feel like it's really all that serious. I have survived this long. I don't feel pain. I don't feel anything. I don't ever feel like anything is wrong with me. Therefore, my kidney disease constantly slips my mind.

Forever Marked

Really, the only time I think about my kidney is when I'm changing in front of a mirror. I see a crooked scar spanning across my stomach. That stupid scar that always made me fold my arms across my stomach when I was at the beach with my friends, or we had that dreaded swimming unit in elementary school. I always wonder what people think when they see my scar. My scar is not subtle. Not even close. It used to be this straight, horizontal line that was maybe five inches long. Apparently scars grow with your body because that sucker is like eight inches now. And when I say crooked, I mean it's *crooked*. It went from looking like someone drew a perfectly straight line with a straight edge to looking like a three-year-old drew branches on a tree. It would be nice if it were straight because it would make me look like I had abs . . . I guess you cannot always get what you want. I have this extreme fear that if I were to ever get pregnant, my scar would tear open. I don't even know if that is possible. I dreamt it once. Now I think about it every now and then. I can picture it slowly pulling apart with the fibers of my skin just holding together by a thread. No matter what any doctor may tell me, one of my biggest fears about having a kid is what carrying a baby could actually do to my body.

Going into my future, I don't know what to expect. Everything is unknown. That's scary, but that's life. I can't imagine my life any different from what it is now. I don't know why. I don't know what lessons I was supposed to learn from having cancer. I don't know why I survived. What good does it do to focus on the "whys" or "why nots" in life? I would like to believe that there is a God somewhere who knew exactly what he was doing; how having cancer and the after-effects from treatment was going to shape me into the person that I will become (because trust me, I am so not there yet). I would like to believe there was some purpose for everything, but I'm just still not sure any of that exists. As reflective as writing about my story has been, I am going to be honest when I say "I'm probably not changing any of my habits right now." I know to be smarter and safer, but I'm only in college for so long. I have the rest of my life to worry. I just do not want to worry right now. I would like to think that is okay. Some days, I would like to pretend like I have absolutely no medical problems, but that will just never be the case. This is my normal.

While Harter's (2013) new normal framework addresses the idea that individuals learn how to adapt to their new life after health disruptions, my experience with Wilm's Tumor and long-term cancer survivorship since the time of my first recollections has been, is, and will continue to be my normal. Rather than a new normal, my long-term cancer survivorship story exists as a to be continued, ever-present, ever-changing normal.

This illness story will never have an ending during my lifetime. There is no "getting over" kidney disease. I do hope the disease does not progress to the point where organ donation and kidney transplant is needed to save my life. I don't know what my future holds or how my past will affect my future. I do know that life is about living for today and being thankful for being right here, right now.

REFLECTION

I wrote this story, not to air out my problems, but to finally, for once, just write everything down on paper. I have had to retell this same old story so many times, I can't even count. Ellis refers to the act of writing out stories that are sometimes difficult to talk about as a "gift to self" and defines the process as a "reflexive attempt to construct meaning in our lives" allowing us to "heal or grow from our pain" (2007, p. 26). While unaware of the need for growth and/or healing when I initially set out to write my story, this truly has been my experience.

Pouring out thoughts and feelings in my health narrative allows me to share my own "suffering, loss, and healing" (Sharf, Harter, Yamasaki, & Haidet, 2011, p. 47) with people I know and complete strangers. I want my story to help anyone suffering with a chronic disease: even one person. Although many do not realize it, reading someone else's health narrative may allow a reader to cope with struggles they face too (Sharf & Vanderford, 2003). If you spent the majority of your life with a chronic illness, never knowing any different, like me, I hope you know that it's okay not to have all of the answers or know every little thing about your illness. It's okay to not always be on top of it. It's okay to sometimes forget that you are living with a chronic condition. It's okay to have some psychological or mental health issues that stem from your health condition. It is okay, as long as you are living the way you want to live. As long as you are happy with where you are at right now—and where you are going.

This process of putting my thoughts and feelings to paper has helped me understand more about why I am the way I am. More than that, I've taken action into my own hands to learn more about my health condition. Before writing this, I really just listened to what the doctors and my parents told me, rather than finding out more for myself.

Lastly, I want to encourage anyone who has a story to tell, to write it. Before writing my own story, I never looked very deeply into stories and studies that were closely related to my health issue and the benefit of storytelling. Doing so has really helped me understand why I am the way that I am. I am not abnormal. My feelings aren't abnormal, and neither are the ways that I react to things. Not only has writing this chapter been therapeutic by helping me learn more about who I am, this process helped me accept who I am. Twenty years after this journey began, it's about time.

NOTES

1. I want to thank my former professor, Jennifer Morey Hawkins, for helping me navigate through the telling and writing of my story, supporting me throughout the process. Without you, I would not even be in the position I am in right now. I am so thankful you believe my story is one to tell.

2. My mother was, and always will be, my rock. Her recollections of the diagnosis and initial treatments were helpful to me in both writing this story and understanding more about myself. Communicating with my mom about everything that has happened to fill in the gaps in my story provided me more appreciation and understanding of who she is as a mother, wife, daughter, sister, and friend.

REFERENCES

American Cancer Society. (n.d.). *Late Effects of Childhood Cancer Treatment*. Retrieved December 05, 2017, from https://www.cancer.org/treatment/chidren-and-cancer/when-your-child-has-cancer/late-effects-of-cancer-treatment.html.

Baltes, P. B., Reese, H. W., & Nesselroade, J. R. (1988). *Introduction to research methods: Life-span developmental psychology*. Hillsdale, NJ: Lawrence Erlbaum.

Derlega, V. J., Winstead, B. A., Folk-Barron, L. (2000). Reasons for and against disclosing HIV-seropositive test results to an intimate partner: A functional perspective. In S. Petronio (Ed.), *Balancing the secrets of private disclosures* (pp. 53–70). New York: Psychology Press.

East L., Jackson D., O'Brien L., & Peters K. (2010). Storytelling: an approach that can help to develop resilience. *Nurse Researcher, 17* (3), 17–25.

Ellingson, L. L. (2017). Realistically ever after: Disrupting dominant cancer narratives within cancer advocacy organizations. *Management Communication Quarterly, 31*, 321–27. doi:10.1177/ 089331891768.9894.

Ellingson, L. L., & Borofka, K. G. E. (2018) Long-term cancer survivors' everyday embodiment. *Health Communication*. Published online. doi: 10.1080/10410236.2018.1550470.

Ellis, C. (2007). Telling secrets, revealing lives: Relational ethics in research with intimate others. *Qualitative Inquiry, 13*, 3–29. doi: 10.1177/1077800406294947.

Fisher, C. L., & Roccotagliata, T. (2017). Interpersonal communication across the life span. In *Oxford Research Encyclopedia of Communication* (pp. 1–35). New York: Oxford University Press. Doi: 10.1093/acrefore/9780190228613.013.201.

Frank, A. (1995). *The wounded storyteller: Body, illness, and ethics*. Chicago, IL: The University of Chicago Press.

Green, D. M., Sklar, C. A., Boice, J. D., Mulvihill, J. J., Whitton, J. A., Stovall, M., & Yasui, Y. (2009). Ovarian failure and reproductive outcomes after childhood cancer treatment:

Results from the childhood cancer survivor study. *Journal of Clinical Oncology, 27*(14), 2374–381. doi: 10.1200/jco.2008.21.1839.

Harter, L. M. (2013). *Imagining new normals: A narrative framework for health communication.* Dubuque, IA: Kendall Hunt Publishing.

Harter, L. M., Japp, P., & Beck, C. S. (2005). Vital problematics of narrative theorizing about health and healing. In L. M. Harter, P. M. Japp, and C. S. Beck (Eds.), *Narratives, health, and healing: Communication theory, research, and practice* (pp. 7–30). Mahwah, NJ: Lawrence Erlbaum Associates, Inc.

Hutson, S. P., Hall, J. M., & Pack, F. L. (2015). Survivor guilt: Analyzing the concept and its contexts. *Advances in Nursing Science, 38*(1), 20–33.

McCreight, B. S. (2004). A grief ignored: narratives of pregnancy loss from a male perspective. *Sociology of Health & Illness, 26*(3), 326–50.

Pennebaker, J. W., & Seagal, J. D. (1999). Forming a story: The health benefits of narrative. *Journal of Clinical Pyschology, 55*(10), 1243–254.

Riessman, C. K. (1993). *Narrative Analysis.* Newbury Park, CA: Sage Publications.

Riessman, C. K. (2003). Analysis of personal narratives. *Inside Interviewing: New Lenses, New Concerns,* 331–45.

Schmidt, S., Petersen, C. & Bullinger, M. (2002). Coping with chronic disease from the perspective of children and adolescents—a conceptual framework and its implications for participation. *Child: Care, Health & Development, 29*(1), 63–75.

Sharf, B. F., Harter, L. M., Yamasaki, J. & Haidet, P. (2011). Narrative turns epic. In T. L. Thompson, R. Parrott, and J. F. Nussbaum (Eds.), *The Routledge handbook of health communication,* 2nd ed. (pp. 36–51). New York: Routledge.

Sharf, B. F. & Vanderford, M. L. (2003). Illness narratives and the social construction of health. In T. L. Thompson, A. Dorsey, K. I. Miller, & R. Parrott (Eds.), *Handbook of health communication* (pp. 9–34). Mahwah, NJ: Lawrence Erlbaum Associates, Inc.

St. Judes Children's Research Hospital. (n.d.). *Wilms Tumor.* (n.d). Retrieved December 05.2017, from https://www.stjude.org/disease/wilms-tumor.html.

Wo, J. Y. & Viswanathan, A. N. (2009) Impact of radiotherapy on fertility, pregnancy, and neonatal outcomes in female cancer patients. *International Journal of Radiation Oncology, Biology, Physics, 73*(5), 1304–312.

Chapter Five

Smoking

A Lifelong Legacy

Ruthann Fox-Hines

PRELUDE: CONFRONTING CONSTRAINTS

The following personal narrative details confrontations with several intersecting challenges: addiction to cigarettes, finding respectful and effective medical treatment, and navigating progressively more severe restrictions associated with respiratory disease inflicted by smoking. These experiences operate at the nexus of three strands of communication research detailed below: the development of smoking behaviors, especially among adolescents; health and disability communication, particularly confronting insensitivity of medical providers and living with debilitating disease; and developing support resources for resilience. This introduction covers the first two areas. The concluding section focuses on resilience and positive communication.

The drive to smoke, especially among adolescents, is fueled by messages that promote smoking as a status symbol. To encourage smoking behavior, tobacco companies promoted cigarettes as signs of maturity, sophistication, and glamor. Gold, Cohen, and Shumate's (2008) examination of cigarette advertisements identifies visual images of "tobacco as a rite of passage into adulthood" (p. 264) and "successful, attractive people use tobacco" (p. 261) as leitmotifs for more than fifty years. During the era that the author initially developed her addiction to smoking, no counter-advertisements warned about the dangers of cigarettes or the long-term consequences of smoking. Paradoxically, the quest for adult independence through smoking eventually would lead to dependence on oxygen to compensate for the effects of lung damage.

The author's experiences also highlight ongoing communication issues in doctor-patient communication, particularly the imperialistic and paternalistic approaches still noticeable among some health professionals. "Competence in communication has been shown to be linked to improved patient outcomes," yet medical school training includes minimal to no formal communication education that could improve the care provider's sensitivity to a patient's emotional needs (Davis, 2010, p. 244). More specifically, patients seek empathic communication that reflects acknowledgment and confirmation of what they are feeling (Bylund & Makoul, 2002). Pecchioni, Wright, and Nussbaum (2005) add that as a patient becomes less functional through age or disease, the risk of miscommunications potentially affecting treatment also rises. The physical and emotional demands of a disability may point to the need for a patient advocate, but a suitable companion may not be available at the time medical care is most needed.

A NARRATIVE OF SMOKING

I smoked my first cigarette at age thirteen. My mother smoked. She died from a variety of cardiovascular issues when I was still twelve. Just months later, I opened the wooden cigarette box on the coffee table by our Duncan Phyfe sofa and there were her Herbert Tareyton, cork-tipped cigarettes. I lit one up, didn't inhale yet—but soon, with the help of friends, learned that grown-up trick.

That was before the cigarette companies began increasing the addictive qualities of their products, so through high school and college, smoking was my way of looking older (I was only twelve when I started high school; I started college at sixteen and graduated at nineteen), but I didn't *feel* addicted. I was sophisticated, accepted by those many years older as one of them. It gave me something to do with my anxious hands. The addiction came later.

Through graduate school at UNC Chapel Hill and an internship at Duke, and then all through a portion of my professional life (I am a licensed counseling psychologist) at USC in Columbia, South Carolina, I smoked and smoked and smoked—up to three packs (sixty cigarettes) a day. So addicted was I, that I couldn't write unless there was a cigarette burning in the ashtray next to me. So addicted, I saved butts and kept them in a tin in case I ran out. So addicted, I was angry with those who talked of black lungs, etc. to scare me about my smoking.

Finally, in the 1990s, the scientific information got through to me[1] and I decided to cut back. That stage lasted for a few years before I could actually say "I want to quit." I finally stopped by switching this addiction to Nicorette gum for almost a decade. Eventually, I weaned myself from the nicotine gum to regular gum, and then eventually grew tired of chewing gum. One of the "gifts" this has given me is an increased patience with folks suffering from addictions. It is not simply a matter of lack of willpower; there is body chemistry involved, and in the case of cigarettes, the cursed cigarette companies knowingly added addictive chemicals to their products.

Unfortunately, the damage had been done.

I must insert that except for the damage smoking did to my body, my health has been rather good. In fact, the birth of my son went relatively well. He was weeks early so I received no anesthetic, and he was breech (bottom first), but I was young and got through it. I recall having read that the average labor lasted twelve hours, so when I experienced excruciating pain and screamed, I would apologize for being such a wimp since I thought it would get even worse in the hours to come. Fortunately, I had counted from the time I went to the hospital and not from the weird little pains I'd had the night before. So, he sat his way into the world soon after a few of my screaming times.

Because I had decided not to nurse, the staff of aides and nurses treated me rather meanly. During the birth, I was torn rather painfully. Healing the stitches, etc. called for the use of some sort of special lamp focused on my vaginal area. The aides never brought the lamp when I was alone in the room; I felt they made sure to bring it when I had company and, thus, the company had to depart early. When my son was brought to me to hold and I unwrapped the blanket, I was yelled at; it wasn't until we got Mark home that I was finally able to count his toes. This was also back in the day when fathers were treated as giant germs, so my husband also was not allowed to hold, see, embrace his son until we were home—away from the disapproving staff.

I have had a life-long battle with eczema starting at about four years of age. It has been a challenge, although not life threatening. I simply learned to live with it with lots of ointments and solutions. There was also the discovery that swimming in the ocean helped, versus swimming in pools, which aggravated it. Currently, I adamantly refuse to even consider the drugs taken internally that the drug companies advertise on TV all the time. The only "C" I got in undergraduate college was in physical education because my eczema was so bad my dermatologist ordered me not to do anything that would make me sweat, so in physical education class that semester all I could do was sit on the sidelines and be a scorekeeper. It pulled my GPA down, but that didn't get in the way of my later getting a masters and PhD from UNC-CH and doing an internship at Duke.

Oh, I almost forgot, I did have decades of major issues with my teeth. In graduate school, I started having abscesses and faced the choice between root canals and extraction; extraction was much cheaper than root canals so since we were poor students, if the tooth was a back tooth, it was extracted at a relatively inexpensive rate. We only spent money for root canals for teeth that were more visible. This problem continued into my professional years when I was finally earning decent money, so I was able to save more teeth. I ended up with root canals in all the remaining teeth. Just another thing to live with. Don't complain, move on. "Others have it worse" are major tenets caregivers often impose on themselves, and care giving was my training. In fact, this aspect of my health became so "normal" I almost forgot to write about it in this chapter.

Dealing with dental stuff was the main time I ever had to resort to pain medication. Way back I found that Demerol was the one drug that worked. All the other drugs dentists tried to prescribe left me with the choice: suffer the excruciating pain or suffer horrible nausea. Pain turned out to be the lesser of the two evils. Dentists seemed afraid to prescribe Demerol due to the increased possibility of addiction, I guess. I'd learned back in graduate school that one or two days on Demerol and I'd be fine, but the doctors of dental surgery (DDS) of later days didn't respect my knowledge of my body and their concern for "addiction" won the day. My only addiction I am aware of is the manufacturer's induced addiction in the cigarettes they produced, and that I smoked.

I feel I have been lucky in the aging arena. I've had no joint problems that so many of my fellow seniors experience as they age. Therefore, I have had no surgeries, replacements, or need for painkillers. Fingers crossed this continues.

For years my body was strong enough to withstand the effects of smoking on my lungs, but in the late nineties, symptoms began to show. The first one I recall was that I found I couldn't last through more than one fast dance without gasping for breath; the second was that uphill hiking became increasingly difficult.

In about 2004, I had a major bronchitis attack, went to a doc-in-the-box (urgent care) and was referred to Dr. Love, a well-known pulmonologist in Columbia, South Carolina. After Xrays, and other tests, he sat down with me and told me that I had emphysema and asthma. And I began to have to use maintenance steroids (Advair) and take drugs for the asthma.

The side effects of the steroids I had and continue to take are a current threat: glaucoma is one result of taking steroids. My eye doctor sees me every six months and thus far the measurements are close, but I am still free of the glaucoma diagnosis. However, now age-related cataracts are a threat, especially since the ophthalmologist is reluctant to do the surgery with my lung issues. He is young, and I can tell he wonders if I will live long enough to risk the surgery. His method of dealing is "Talk to your pulmonologist and see what he thinks." Interesting how even doctors often find end-of-life issues difficult to discuss with patients.

The steroids also can have a very negative effect on my bones. My female gynecologist has, for years, prescribed hormones that can help prevent/slow down bone deterioration even before the steroids, since I am considered rather thin. I read the pertinent research and wrote her a letter for my file saying I wanted the hormones and realized the risks. One of the things I've had to deal with in small and sometimes large ways are male physicians who do not respect my knowledge of my own body. I have had encounters with some male doctors who had the "I am God, do not question me" syndrome, but more about that later. My female gynecologist respected my research and my knowledge of my body and has agreed that, for me, the hormones are worth it.

Before I forget or get back to the focal health issues, COPD and asthma, I want to share my story about the "God" doctor. I'd had a typical bladder infection. We women are very familiar with these and know what is needed: a specific medication for urinary-tract pain, an antibiotic Rx for the infection, and because antibiotics too often cause yeast infections in women, an anti-yeast Rx. I went to a "doc-in-the-box" and told the doctor I have a bladder infection and need the usual prescriptions. After confirming my diagnosis via my peeing bloody urine in a cup, he wrote two of the three prescriptions, one for pain and one antibiotic.

When I went to get those filled, the female pharmacist reminded me that earlier I had purchased an over-the-counter version of the pain medication and shouldn't use both, so we didn't bother with that prescription. I am so thankful for the pharmacists I know and who, I think because of my appreciation for them, remember me and show me their skills and extra care.

I didn't notice the anti-yeast prescription was missing until I was at the pharmacy. So, the next day, I returned to the "doc-in-the-box" facility and told the receptionist, "All I need is for you to give the MD this note" on which I had written the name of the anti-yeast prescription I needed.

The receptionist returned to me and rather sheepishly said, "The doctor will not write the prescription." *What?! I guess I need to talk with the MD.* The doctor was not the one from the previous day. He was an Indian doctor who screamed at me, "I will *not* fill this prescription!" I tried to explain to him that all the medical folks I'd dealt with understood the need for women to get anti-yeast medication when they are put on an antibiotic. He glared at me and yelled, "Well, get one of those doctors to write it for you!" And when I started to re-explain, he yelled again, "You *get the infection* and then I'll write the prescription!"

Luckily, I am not easily daunted and have learned to advocate for myself. I went online, found contact administrators, and emailed and called the directors to report how I had been treated, with total lack of respect, etc. I suspect that doctor had a history of treating women in general that way, even the employees at the clinic. Because of my calls, very quickly I was told that the first doctor was there and would write the prescription I needed, and I could pick it up that day. I did lodge a formal complaint against Dr. Patel, but my energy was elsewhere (recovering from the painful infection) as far as seeing if he ended up getting a reprimand.

What really disturbs me about that encounter is the way some doctors treat women; I was capable of advocating for myself, but what if all the women that doctor dealt with were not as capable? Or, what about when I might be less capable and there are medical personnel such as him practicing medicine?

Even after the asthma and COPD diagnoses, I did OK for several years. My partner, Roy, and I enjoyed lots of hiking, especially along the Blue Ridge Parkway in Virginia, North Carolina, and Georgia. For years, even after the diagnoses, I walked three to five miles a day, but gradually I had the need to begin finding routes that had less and less of a grade to deal with. He would even investigate and plan routes where the incline would be sharpest as we were heading home and downhill.

After about 2008, Roy and I began to find even easier hiking trails for us. He would do the more strenuous on his own, but we kept going. I kept going.

The debilitation was slow but steady until 2015. In late June, we went on a cruise on the Danube River, and for the touring, I'd take the easy tours and Roy would do the normal tours. I loved the trip. Roy developed a difficult sinus infection, and the last part of the trip was not pleasant. The Budapest airport was a crazy, misrun, crowded, horrible place. My immune system went down, and within a couple of days back home in Columbia, Roy was rushing me to the urgent clinic. Despite having had two different pneumonia shots, I managed to pick up a strain of pneumonia that wasn't covered by the American shots.

The doctor there was so frightened by my oxygen levels, he told Roy, "The only way she is leaving here is in an ambulance." So, he called an ambulance and I was rushed to Palmetto-Baptist (I chose that one because Dr. Love was affiliated with it). I was conscious the whole time. Part of my brain kicked into "observer" mode, noting that this was my first ride as the sick person in an ambulance and it was serious enough that they had the siren going. At Baptist, the emergency-room medical doctor, who must have been Baptist, asked me all those stupid questions they ask. One was, "How much do you drink?" I answered that I had two to three glasses of champagne every day. I think they are trained to double whatever the number people say they drink, so he got very concerned. "You know you cannot drink in the hospital." *Duh, yes.* "You may get the DTs." *Oh, Christ, he's worried about me and delirium tremors (DTs) and I'm dying from lack of oxygen!*

I spent the next ten days in the intermediate intensive care unit hooked up to all sorts of monitors and tethered so tightly that I couldn't even get to the bathroom. I had to use a rolling potty that was placed by the bed. For the first several days, there was always a technician observing. No semblance of dignity allowed.

I felt like I was in the middle of a comedy routine. At least a "cover our asses routine." Because I'd traveled abroad, the administrators of the hospital decided I might have tuberculosis, so some of my blood was taken for testing and until the results could be reported, my room was in semi-quarantine. There was a giant machine hauled in to suck air out of the room, and visitors and staff had to don masks. Since I was on an inhaler, making myself understood was not easy; then with the staff all wearing masks, we had quite a circus trying to communicate. It took a few days before I was declared "safe."

In addition to having to poop with an audience, there were many minor indignities including the required garb, a hospital gown. I am at the most about 110 pounds; the gown I was assigned was an XL which fell off me in many directions. I befriended the nurses and aides by listening and mainly using humor to get through situations, so when I asked for a smaller gown they went on a real search. It seems that to save money, the hospital only had that one size. For the duration of my stay I was constantly tugging my gown to maintain a tiny modicum of modesty.

As I got better, when I coughed a lot, my bladder leaked a few drops. I mentioned that I would like Depends to help me handle the problem. I had to sign a release so Roy could bring me in some Depends-like product. Hospital administrators had to protect us patients from terrible outside dangers, or were they annoyed that I didn't want them to provide the diapers at probably fifty dollars a pair. Luckily my bladder control improved and I didn't need them.

During the last two-thirds of my stay, there was my bag-lady period. Although too many nursing technicians were waking me every hour during the nights, when signing in with their supervisor Mrs. Green and conversing during charting, they were not available during the day to bring me things. So I took to hoarding stuff that I needed: tissues, a tissue box that I used as a mini trashcan since the only trashcan in the room was a giant one far from the bed (with all the machines monitoring me, there was no room for a trashcan near the bed), hand wipes (I only was bathed twice during the nine-day stay), drinks (ice and water and ginger ale were not that easy to obtain), protein bars and cookies so I could have something to eat besides the mostly not-so-appealing food, a comb, glasses, ChapStick, and other essentials.

All items were stored on the bedside tray table and it felt like a version of a homeless woman's grocery bag. I became very protective of all the items I had gathered in it. The nurses and techs soon learned to be respectful of my little "trashcan" and the other items that made life tethered in a bed easier. I had them laughing with my reference to myself as "The Bag Lady of the

IICU." I'd been sort of a slow learner about using a smart phone, but I sure did appreciate the texting aspect while stuck in the hospital bed; I could use it to let Roy or my son Mark know things I'd like them to bring to me.

Roy was in town during my hospitalization, but because of the agony of his sinus infection, he mainly had to stay away to take care of himself. My son was also in town but hanging out in a small hospital room wasn't that conducive to his getting work done on his computer, so most of the time I was alone. Good preparation for my recovery at home. Roy had to leave the day after I got out of the hospital, my son stayed for several more days, and then I was on my own.

The inhalation therapist in charge of that aspect of my release told me that she intended for me to fail her test, so I could have Medicare cover at-home oxygen. She succeeded (I failed), and I was sent home attached to a tank of oxygen by a very important thing called a cannula. Not long after arriving home, a man arrived with more tanks like those used by scuba divers plus a giant (twenty-four-hour) one, and a machine that produced oxygen, which he delivered and set up.

I gradually gathered strength at home and within a couple of months I was able to accompany Roy to a house we rent each late spring on Sunset Beach, North Carolina.

That fall (2017) I resumed my commute between Columbia, South Carolina, where I have a private practice as a psychologist and Greensboro, North Carolina, where Roy is a professor at UNCG. I had to keep the oxygen nearby just in case. So, when I traveled, friends would load up or unload my car in Columbia and Roy would handle the unloading or loading in Greensboro. Unfortunately, being in Greensboro became more and more of a problem because my allergies to cats grew worse and worse and Roy's cats were/are his *children*, so I had to be the one to clear out.

March 2018 was the last time I was in Greensboro. My stamina had gone way down, and my breathing issues had increased significantly. I packed up. Roy loaded the car, and I managed to get back to Columbia where I nearly collapsed. I kept going for a couple of days before I was so bad off I had to dial 911 and ended up back at Baptist Hospital ER. No questions this time about alcohol or concern for DTs.

This time I ended up spending two days in a windowless room in the emergency services area because the hospital was full of folks with breathing problems. My sense of humor got me through a lot of the difficulties of hospitalization. In fact, I still have some selfies I took when hidden under complex breathing equipment. Somehow several friends heard of my situation and came to the ER and visited. Eventually, my partner (from Greensboro, North Carolina) and my son (from Chicago) were able to also come and be with me.

In retrospect, I suspect I was close to death. After all, being able to breathe *is* a large part of being alive. I'm grateful that it was all somewhat surreal: emergency medical technicians, another ambulance with a siren going, ER, neighbors' faces, friends leaving work to come be with me, all sorts of breathing equipment in place. I never lost consciousness. I think that was a good sign some oxygen must have been getting to my brain.

When they did find me a room, it was a *good room*, almost a suite on the oncology floor. It was on the top floor with a very nice view of a Columbia cityscape. There was plenty of room for Roy and Mark to set all their electronics so they could work while being with me. Unlike my first hospitalization, my tethering wasn't quite as restrictive. I was able to use the bathroom alone, and have privacy. I remembered my Bag Lady persona and was very careful about keeping my stuff safe. I also expanded my electronic repertoire to a tablet, which was great for emails, etc. so I could feel connected to others. Since I wasn't in enforced isolation, for the first time I could also have more visitors, and that felt great.

Oh, the term for this "incident" is an "exacerbation" of my COPD condition. Treatment equaled *lots* of steroids: ingested in pill form, given intravenously, and administered as an inhalant every four hours around the clock. Rest, of course, was also absolutely needed. With movement also important as with the first time, I would switch from the bed to a chair for the good part of the daylight hours.

As with the first time in the hospital, my appetite was zero, so I told the food folks to get me lots of liquid protein and I forced that down as much as possible. Eventually, I had a hankering for real food. "Product placement" in this story: I craved Bojangles dark meat fried chicken and dirty rice. Roy or Mark brought me all I could eat. The first time in the hospital I went down to about 98 pounds. This time I stayed a pound or two above 100 pounds.

I'd already had practice at recovering at home; although this time I had to adjust to using oxygen 24/7. Before I'd been able to do without oxygen while sleeping or resting and "only" needed it when I was active; this time my doctor was very firm about my using it around the clock.

Adjusting to being tethered to an oxygen machine was a bit of a challenge. I did get a long tether, about fifty feet of tubing. Then that thing you see in TV programs when folks are in the hospital, a cannula, which is a softer tube that goes over the ears and has tiny tubes that go in each nostril. Again, one size fits all, but I lucked out and the ones I have work OK. Somehow, I still want to call it "cannoli" (the plural form of wonderful Italian dessert. A much more pleasant word).

Using the tether, I developed great empathy for dogs on long leads and how they get tangled around trees or bushes. My kitchen has two doors, one from the hall and one into the dining room. The hall leads either to the back of the house and bedroom and the room my oxygen machine is in. Or the hall leads to the front of the house and the living room. Picture this: I walk from the hall into the kitchen, take something into the dining room and the doorbell rings so I go to answer it in the living room. Ouch! Yank, harsh pull on my ears and nose and I am stopped. The tether ran out, so I must back up into the dining room, go back through the kitchen into the hall, and then go to answer the front door. I think I may be a slower learner than my canine friends since I am six months into the tether and I still experience the Ouch! Yank, harsh pull on my ears and nose.

I used to enjoy the power of thunderstorms; now they are a source of dread. Will they cause a power outage and cut me off from the oxygen my machine provides? Of course, I have some tanks, like the tanks divers use, that I keep as back-ups in case of outages, but the threat still is: Will the ones I have be enough to last through a long outage? The power company has me on a list but provides no guarantees that they will get to me as soon as I might need. Also, the tanks are heavy and managing them is not easy.

As I became more and more dependent on oxygen machines, I became more and more house bound, except when someone else could haul the tanks around for me. Medicare covers the in-house machine and the tanks, but not portable oxygen machines. I finally went into my savings and came up with the thousands of dollars for a portable machine. It has given me a degree of freedom I didn't have. However, the portable machine's delivery system is different from the in-house machine. The in-house provides a constant flow of oxygen. The portable one provides oxygen as a pulse and adjusting to the difference has not been easy. At first, I added to the difficulty with anxiety about "doing it right." That only made breathing more difficult. Finally, I decided to befriend the portable machine as a friend that accompanies me on adventures out of the house, albeit the adventures are usually trips to the grocery store or drugstore or bank, but I am getting out of the house. My machine is now "My Buddy," and My Buddy and I go to lunch with friends, do errands, go to doctors, etc.

Because this latest exacerbation was such a significant one, I could no longer avoid facing at least some of the details of living with a progressive and terminal disease. While Roy and Mark were here, I got my friend/attorney to come by and redo my will, all those power of attorney things, etc. The four of us sat in my living room and everything was wide open. She explained things to my son and to Roy and helped the three of us make decisions. A few days later, she brought her paralegal and a woman who has an office in her building (she is a social worker who is also a well-known fiction author) to act as witnesses for all the paperwork. After the witnesses left the attorney and I had visiting time. She doesn't work with me on a clock.

Roy had to get back to his university work, so he had to leave and return to Greensboro before my son had to leave. He could do some of his work via his computer and phone. Mark was amazing in taking command of the whole situation. He set me up with an aide service, grocery service, etc., etc., etc. He inventoried all of my major paperwork. I made arrangements with my friend/colleague, Toby, to shred any client information that might be left when I die.

The whole thing was a very *in my face* experience with *I am going to die*—not this very moment, but . . .

In the beginning, Mark set me up with a service that provided aides 24/7. I didn't need that (at least not now; later in my illness, most likely), but it really helped to have an aide for three hours in the morning each day helping with meals and things I wasn't yet strong enough to do. Three of the aides sent to me were wonderful, going the extra bit to make my life easier; one was putting in her time; and one was a very stressed, unhappy woman. Since I am a psychologist, I have learned that listening is usually the best way to let people know I respect them. This did help a lot and I learned a lot about life on the poverty line. All of the women worked at least one full-time and one part-time job. One worked a full-time job and two part-time jobs. Most were raising children on their own or caring for ailing parents at home. I get so angry with wealthy or simply well-off folks who denigrate the poor as lazy and worthless.

I had some fun times with the aides. One went beyond her duties and moved a trundle bed from the guest room and set it up in the dining room so I could have a rest station there where I also have a TV up on a high shelf. She moved things with such ease and when I commented, she posed and said, "these are Mommy arms!" Another helped me bring out spring/summer clothes and put away fall/winter stuff. She loved shoes and spent any spare money on shoes, so she taught me how to store shoes and fit more into the space available. We worked together. Well, I'd sit and say what I needed, and she would do it, but we laughed.

My last aide (until the next exacerbation) was Lillian, an older woman who worked full time at a house for the mentally disabled and then came to me from noon to four in the afternoon twice a week. I had grown stronger and could do much more like fix simple meals, but I was not strong enough to do such things as sorting through "treasures" to simplify and cull down possessions. She is such a beautiful, gentle soul. I hope that when I need aides again, she may still be working.

One of the issues of aging and illness is the negative effects of isolation. Too often older people retreat from the world, and the research clearly shows, isolation is deadly.[2] With my illness, I must retreat to some degree, at least from crowded places, because if I catch a cold or, God forbid, the flu, it could hasten my approach to the Pearly Gates. So, I have to negotiate a balance between getting out of the house, maintaining strong connections with friends/colleagues/family, and avoiding exposure to viruses and bad forms of bacteria.

One thing I've done is be very open with friends about the disease and my vulnerability and they warn me, or they alter their plans to visit if they have been exposed to dangerous germs. I do not go to Sunday services at church because the pews are too often filled with hacking folks who have dragged themselves there with their sick children. I do not go to evening movies, etc. I keep a mask handy just in case.

Because I am a psychologist who has preached for years about the importance of a support system, I work very hard to maintain and keep building a healthy support system. I have friends who I can call on when things are difficult, friends I can have fun with, friends I can share political and professional concerns with, etc. A giant mistake too many people make is selecting one other human being, often the spouse, and designating that human being as *the* support system. One person does not equal a "system." It is way past what is humanly possible for one person to be that in entirety for another.

I also realized it is *my responsibility* to develop and maintain, for as long as I can, my support system. It is not my partner's responsibility. It is not my son's responsibility. It is not my friends' responsibility to take care of me. They have lives, and I know I need to respect that.

It is my job, and I do it by keeping in touch with folks via email and a little via the phone. I do not text except in situations such as being in the hospital or picking someone up at an airport. I have strong feelings about the phone being an invasive instrument. I can call you when it is convenient for me but frequently not convenient for you. With email, I can write when it works for me. You can read what I write when it works for you. I can read what you write when it works for me. Neither of us are at the beck and call of the other. I also actually write letters to some folks. That art is dying, but I've decided that I will keep it going until I die.

I have clients (yes, despite my illness, I still see clients—no new ones, but I enjoy working with my long-term clients) whose parents demand attention and service and use guilt trips to manipulate their children and friends. I do my very best to avoid anything that hints of that type of behavior in my situation. I see the pain it causes my clients. Instead, I take on the responsibility of reaching out to friends for small services or for companionship, fun, etc. I keep a list of folks and I try very hard not to call on any one neighbor or friend too often for an errand or chore.

Two neighbors are very kind and email me when they are going to go shopping and ask if they can pick something up for me. I keep a list of things that are getting low so when they call I can ask for a couple of items. I have gotten strong enough that I can, using "*My* Buddy" the portable oxygen machine, go to a grocery store or drugstore. I did learn the hard way about how much was OK to buy. One excursion to Publix found me feeling particularly good. I shopped and shopped, then used the "no tip please" carry out to car service. Everything was great until I got home, and realized I had to get all those groceries into the house by myself. I did it, but it took about an hour because I would get two bags in and then have to sit and breathe and get my oxygen levels up above the danger point (85 percent) before I could go back out and bring in two more bags. I now am more cautious in terms of what I shop for and what I ask others to get for me. I leave "heavy" items such as a half-gallon of milk or canned goods for when neighbors shop for me. I stick to lighter items such as produce or bread.

When I was first out of the hospital, a friend, colleague, and neighbor, Sally, took on the responsibility of arranging folks to come visit me so I wouldn't be isolated. I provided her a list of friends and colleagues. After several weeks, two months or so, I was well enough to do that for myself. Now I make sure to regularly set up lunch dates, inviting folks over for happy hour times, and other social events. I find the loneliest times are the weekends since most people have families, errands, events, and chores that absorb most of their weekend time. Plus, that's often the time they can sleep in, indulging themselves a little. So, I plan for weekends to be "work" times to do such things as this, writing. Once in a while I am pleasantly surprised by a friend who drops by just to see me.

A very recent addition to my strategies in living with this disease is a collapsible transport wheelchair, a very lightweight one. Since I do not weigh a whole lot, most healthy adults can push me around in it. While the portable oxygen makes getting out of the house possible, it doesn't make up for my lack of stamina and my breathing issues when I walk around. Going out in nature, going to craft fairs, going to festivals, and going to museums were all things that were beyond my ability to do. With someone pushing me in the wheelchair, all of those are again possibilities. My shrinking world has expanded. The first excursion out was with Roy pushing me on 2.5 miles of boardwalk in the Congaree National Park, a beautiful swampland not far from Columbia, South Carolina.

Most of my adult life, I have been an activist, a feminist, and antiwar protestor. Now it is too complicated to get to meetings, and marching is not a possibility. I can still sit at a computer and write. I stay an activist via donating what I can *and* writing emails and Facebook posts especially.

During my whole professional life, I spoke in front of groups of a few to those of hundreds on topics of mental and physical health, interpersonal communication, stress management, and burnout prevention. Now I must really listen to all the things I taught and heed my own advice. I did try to do that all along, but this illness/disease forces the issue. I still try to be there for others in my very small private practice and via writing. Although I still have dreams of running workshops that expand from a dozen folks in a room to hundreds of folks in many different rooms. Guess my *busy-busy* approach to life didn't drop away even though my ability to be busy-busy did.

So, this is where I am now. Living each day as fully as I can. Being Ruthann as fully as I can. I used to be a *participant*-observer in my life. Now I am a participant-*observer*.

CODA: RESILIENCE WITHIN A SHRINKING WORLD

One of the most important threads in the author's narrative is the role that positive communication plays in building resilience during a lifespan affected by debilitating illness. The progressive constrictions on her breathing inflict further constraints on personal mobility and on interpersonal relationships that had been sustained by shared activities. Disabilities can disrupt social networks that had not previously accounted for the changes wrought by illness. Therefore, innovative ways to maintain connectivity become imperative (Reznik, 2019). Tethered by the oxygen tube that provides her lifeline, the author—by nature and profession a caregiver—must increasingly find within herself the resources to explore her personal agency amid a shrinking world. As Kellett (2017) notes in his personal narrative of progressive loss of vision, developing self-advocacy skills prove essential in managing one's own well-being. Abundant research documents the positive emotional and physical health impact of supportive communication (Pecchioni, Wright, & Nussbaum, 2005). As well as in fostering a sense of self-efficacy in the face of setbacks (Burleson & MacGeorge, 2002), hence the centrality in the preceding narrative of reaffirming communication with friends and caregivers.

As Beck and Socha (2015) observe, relational networks play a crucial role in coping with and countering the debilitating effects of adversity. Communication with others not only can provide hope and encouragement, it also prevents self-absorption that can spiral into negativity and withdrawal. These ongoing interactions energize the "process of effective negotiation, adaptation or resource management in times of stress and trauma" that characterizes resilience, counteracting the immersion in distress, sorrow, or other chronically negative emotions that generate "psychache" (Ohana, Golander, & Barak, 2014, pp. 929–30).

Recognizing the constant potential for isolation, the narrator has grown to appreciate the activities still possible despite increasingly restricted mobility: increasing her physical range through a wheelchair, appreciating her interactions with others (in person or electronically), maintaining a sense of humor that puts suffering in perspective (DiCioccio, 2015), and advocating for social causes by writing instead of marching or demonstrating. These adaptations enact resilience as "an ongoing struggle to create and sustain the new normal that comes from recognition that life cannot be the same as it was before" (Buzzanell & Shenoy-Packer, 2015, p. 150). Pushing back against the multiple moments of marginalization she experiences as a patient, as a woman, and as a person with limited mobility, the author affirms her capacity for agency amid her contracting world.

NOTES

1. In a study of smoking initiation among twelve-to-thirteen year olds, a recent study notes: "Growing evidence on how quickly ND [nicotine dependency] symptoms can manifest after the first puff supports treating the first puff as a clinical emergency necessitating intervention to prevent long-term smoking" (p. 4). Sylvestre, M. P., Hanusaik, N., Berger, D., Dugas, E., Pbert, L., Winickoff, J., & O'Loughlin, J. L. (2018). A tool to identify adolescents at risk of cigarette smoking initiation. *Pediatrics, 142*(5), 1–10. Apparently the tobacco industry funded studies to prove a genetic basis for nicotine addiction so that the responsibility for smoking could be deflected away from the tobacco companies. A detailed analysis appears in Gundle, K. R., Dingel, M. J., & Koenig, B. A. (2010). 'To prove this is the industry's best hope': Big tobacco's support of research on the genetics of nicotine addiction. *Addiction, 105*(6), 974–83.

2. Almost fifty years of studies converge on this finding. Social isolation correlates strongly with negative health outcomes for seniors, but social support can reverse or slow many of these effects. See Tomaka, J., Thompson, S., & Palacios, R. (2015). The relation of social isolation, loneliness, and social support to disease outcomes among the elderly. *Community Development Journal, 50*(3), 359–384. The detrimental effects of loneliness encompass cognitive functioning, emotional well-being, and physical health. See Masi, C. M., Chen, H.-Y., Hawkley, L. C., & Cacioppo, J. T. (2011). A meta-analysis of interventions to reduce loneliness. *Personality and Social Psychology Review, 15*(3), 219–66.

REFERENCES

Beck, G. A., & Socha, T. J. (2015). *Communicating hope and resilience across the lifespan*. New York: Peter Lang.

Burleson, B. R., & MacGeorge, E. L. (2002). Supportive communication. In M. L. Knapp & J. A. Daly (Eds.), *Handbook of interpersonal communication* (3rd ed.). Thousand Oaks, CA: Sage.

Buzzanell, P. M., & Shenoy-Packer, S. (2015). Resilience, work, and family communication across the lifespan. In G. A. Beck & T. J. Socha (Eds.), *Communicating hope and resilience across the lifespan* (pp. 138–55). New York: Peter Lang.

Bylund, C. L., & Makoul, G. (2002). Empathic communication and gender in the physician-patient encounter. *Patient Education and Counseling, 48*(3), 207–16.

Davis, D. L. (2010). Simple but not always easy: Improving doctor-patient communication. *Journal of Communication in Healthcare, 3*(3/4), 240–45.

DiCioccio, R. L. (2015). 'We could sure use a laugh': Building hope and resilience through humorous communication. In G. A. Beck & T. J. Socha (Eds.), *Communicating hope and resilience across the lifespan* (pp. 34–52). New York: Peter Lang.

Gold, A. L., Cohen, E. L., & Shumate, M. (2008). Proscriptive models and evidence in anti-smoking advertising. *Health Communication, 23*(3), 259–69.

Kellett, P. M. (2017). *Patienthood and communication: A personal narrative of eye disease and vision loss*. New York: Peter Lang.

Ohana, I., Golander, H., & Barak, Y. (2014). Balancing psychache and resilience in aging Holocaust survivors. *International Psychogeriatrics, 26*(6), 929–34.

Pecchioni, L. L., Wright, K. B., & Nussbaum, J. F. (2005). *Life-span communication*. Mahwah, N.J.: Lawrence Erlbaum.

Reznik, R. R. (2019). Narratives of patient experience: Benefits for multiple audiences. In P. M. Kellett (Ed.), *Narrating patienthood: Engaging diverse voices on health, communication, and the patient experience* (pp. 3–16). Lanham, MD: Lexington.

Part II

Middles

Chapter Six

Through the Glass Darkly

How We Fill a Diagnosis with Meaning

Laura Hope-Gill

One point on Earth is still believed to bear the earth's original crust. At 4.4 billion years old, this small patch of stone lies within the Canadian Shield spanning the northeast of Ontario and across into Québec. Lowered mountains form a complex shoreline unified underwater and, above-surface, thirty thousand islands. Although the region is not fully mapped, the Canadian Group of Seven and Tom Thomson have documented portions in vibrant, innovative brushstrokes giving Canada its first genuine artistic expression and pallet separate from British landscape heritage. In the Northwoods forests, small pools of rainwater collect on beds of bright mosses. Birches peel summer away in thin strips that flutter in the wind. Solitary elms yet grow healthily on stone islands, protected from west winds by jack pine, or nothing at all. *Nothing at all* is a part of the landscape as well there—vast swathes of it stretch upon the horizon between rocks and trees. Uninterrupted. White caps lap against solidified ribbons of rose quartz encased in granite. The water's blue seems to deepen the sky, and at night the stars swim. Across it all, for sixty million years, the cry of the loon has traveled.

I have loved its song throughout childhood. I have canoed out in early mornings and stowed my paddle to drift on mist arising from the waves and waited, and having heard it, I have echoed. I have gaged the quality of my own humanity by whether or not a loon would answer me, a way of sounding my connection to this earth. My laugh to its laugh. My slow cry to its slow cry. Even when one was washed up on to the Siesta Key sand in winter plumage, my mother brought it home to recuperate, and I sang to it in its cardboard box, and it sang back. I have been the whisperer of loons in the most precious untold narrative of summers in Muskoka and Parry Sound and even winters in Florida. I have been the one to stop everyone from talking so we could all hear it when it spoke. And it was the loon that betrayed me when I first was going deaf.

My mother noticed my deafness first and after a week of observation confronted me. I was visiting at her cottage on Georgian Bay. The cottage is a small, genuine cottage built the way cottages used to be built: with one common room and kitchen and very small bedrooms behind doors coming off from it. It is necessary to describe this because now people are building much larger cottages with grand atriums and huge bedrooms. My mom and stepdad's cottage is pretty much the same design as the one my mother and father used to rent down the highway a bit in Muskoka. This new cottage is north of Parry Sound and takes an hour of driving on dirt road and eventually bare rock to get to. Situated on a point facing west, it is a magnificent place to watch the sun set.

My ninety-four-year-old grandmother, Nanny, was with us too. A lifelong lover of the Northwoods, she still paddled a canoe then sipped tea on the small porch. Poppee had died eight years before in 1993, and she felt his presence in the wilderness. She also felt it in her nursing home where she insisted on staying through Christmases, their anniversary. "Jim knows how to find me here," she would say when we invited her to Asheville. Sipping tea beside her, I would swear Poppee was with us too. The sunlight on Georgian Bay feels like breath on July afternoons. Everything reflects blue from the water. Sitting on the porch with Nanny, I watched the calm bay. Occasionally, a snapping turtle popped up its head. A water snake scaled the surface then vanished in the reeds along the shore. Birch trees stock-still in the miniature forests of the north, their leaves unmoved on the windless day. I held Nanny's hand. In silence we sat, observing water, stone, and sky in all their wind-hushed stillness. My mother joined us, tea cup in hand, legs propped up on the bench. A whole afternoon passed like that, the three of us absorbed into the scenery, breathing it in as though we were fish returned to water. We held hands when we were not sipping tea. The three of us were together, and we sat in the silence, allowing all that surrounded us to melt into us, to become imprinted by us so that moment would last forever.

That evening we were seated at the wooden table my step-dad, Dick, a retired fish and wildlife biologist and now wood carver, had made.

Mom said, "You can't hear the loons."

I found the statement horribly offensive. I had always heard the loons. The loons were not talking.

"There are no loons," I said as I poured water from the blue summer-plastic pitcher. All the blue summer plastic in the cottage held the story of the cottage's purchase. Mom and Dick had spent a week in a rented, run-down cottage in Algonquin Park, then asked a real estate agent to show them what was available. It was love at first sight for this cottage that would be sold fully furnished so they made an offer. On the day before closing, my mother asked the owners if they would leave the blue summer plastic and cutlery in the kitchen. This tipped the wife into a pre-facto state of seller's remorse, and she withdrew the contract. To assuage, my mother and step-dad offered to let them use the cottage for two weeks for the next three summers. This agreement was written into the contract, and for the first three summers of their ownership, Mom and Dick vacated the premises for two weeks in July and traveled to Nova Scotia or rode the Polar Express. The blue plastic is still there, twenty years later.

"There!" My mother actually shouted. "You don't hear that do you?"

Trying to hear a loon is something I had never learned to do. The sound had just come into me. To try to hear a loon, press your lower jaw up against the rest of your skull. Squint your eyes as though vision has something to do with this. Focus your mind on thin air pretending it is a net that will catch some sonic thing flying through it like a gnat. Remember the call as you know it in your bones, then press that memory upon the present moment to make it real again. And fail. Fail terribly. Fail in front of everyone at the table, in front of all that summer plastic.

"Do you hear a loon?" I asked Dick, who nodded.

"And you hear a loon?" I asked Mom.

"There, again!" she said. Challenging me. Not out of any sort of meanness but challenging me with encouragement. She was giving me the answer to the test of whether or not my hearing was off. She was also possibly inviting me to lie so we did not have to follow the path my not hearing a loon could lead us down.

Noting the cry of the loon is a main feature in the Katharine Hepburn and Henry and Jane Fonda masterpiece *On Golden Pond.* "The loons, Henry, listen to the loons," Hepburn says shakily, her age never defeating her magnificence and, if anything, only augmenting it. We used to laugh at ourselves because that is exactly what we would do when the loon pair on the bay just past our own, a little curve within the immense Franklin Island, called out. We would hear the call and stop everything like it's the one sound in the world worth stopping everything for. Haunting. Long. Primordial. As old as the blue whale's call, the loon's call is the closest we can get to hearing the song of time itself. There are three loon calls I can do, only three that I know of. The first is like a dot-dash in Morse-code or a quarter note and whole note in sheet music. Only it's very long, like when the whole note lasts four or five measures and then fades into the wilderness beyond the shore of silence.

The second call is the maniacal laugh that won the birds synonymy with a form of madness: a complete loon, the loony bin. This call begins in the back of the throat then rises like a soprano hitting the highest G in a cathedral in rhythmic steps all very quickly. To make this sound, let your mouth make an ever-widening shape and let your neck bob for the highest beats. Then you repeat it. You repeat it and repeat it and repeat it. In the Pacific Northwest where I lived in my little cabin and ventured into the town of Port Angeles only to teach basic education four hours four days of the week, I once sat at my little 1950's diner table writing and looked up and saw about eighty loons on Sequim Bay out my window. They do this. They have parties, and at the parties they call out in this joyful sound and dance on the water, breast to breast with wings in full extension. They check in like that, and that call is what brings them all together.

It was easy for my mother to see something was wrong when she heard the loon that evening and I did not. She even waited through a series of cries and watched me continue setting the table with the blue summer plastic now well-scratched from so many trips through a dishwasher so old I am surprised there are not Roman numerals on the dial. The loon called out. I set the forks and knives. The loon called again. I poured water from the blue pitcher into the blue glasses. Then my mother spoke, and my world began to change.

My mother's first hope was that my inability to hear loons stemmed from sinus trouble. Side by side with my grandmother after dinner, we sat at the dining room table my step-dad had made, and we logged a good (precious) hour with our heads over bowls of steaming water under towels, trying to empty our nasal passages of various gunk. Nanny had much more gunk than I did, and she just kept winning the nose-blowing game, reaching and reaching for tissue after tissue.

"I don't know why she's making us do this," Nanny said to me under the privacy of our little steam tent. "Seems a terrible waste of time." She blew her nose, winning again.

I was clearly the loser. Hardly a sniffle. That did not stop Mom, though. Every night for the next two weeks, Nanny and I steamed together. When I returned home, I asked my doctor for some nasal decongestant, nose spray, anything to help a condition my mother was certain I had. I squirted Flonase for five weeks. And while there are no loons of note in Asheville, North Carolina, my mother continued to witness signs that Flonase was not the answer.

The week before my teaching started at Christ School for Boys and Mom's teaching started at Haw Creek Elemetary, Mom called and asked me to meet her for lunch while she prepared her learning skills lab. I suggested a restaurant, but she said she wanted to keep working but was hungry. I packed sandwiches and little glass bottles of apple juice. Instead of finding my mother hard at work unpacking her boxes of teaching supplies, I found her sitting with another teacher. On the table there was a black machine with lights, some on some off, and a set of headphones. There was also a chart of some sort, and the teacher my mom talked with held a pen.

"What's going on, Mom?"

"Well, honey, this is Jan. Jan's the speech therapist here, and she wants to test your hearing."

"It's just sinuses, Mom. The Flonase will work soon."

Jan cut in. "It will just take about fifteen minutes." I don't know if Jan knew that she was an instrument of ambush and deceit, a violation of long trust between mother and daughter. I sat down and placed the paper bag of lunch on the floor. I put the headphones on and rattled off responses each time I heard a beep or tone and said words Jan said to me back to Jan. I was hungry. I wanted my sandwich. I was thirsty. I wanted my juice. Jan's face as she examined the chart on the paper then put down her pen revealed concern not only for me but for her friend, my mom. She was about to change both our lives with her report.

My mother came over to the table where Jan broke the news that "There's something wrong, and it's serious." I needed to go to an audiologist. This held no meaning for me at the time. I let the words stick to me like sandspurs but not enter me like needles. It was something that was interesting, an interesting development, certainly not something that would become a part of my life. It would be treated and taken away. It was a hassle, that is all. I'd double up on Flonase and spend more time under a tea towel and over steam like I had with Nanny. Normally, my mother's face is easy for me to read. So is her voice. I have always been able to read through to a truth she's hiding. But on that day, I could not, or did not know what possible truths existed. She knew better than I did what the marks on the audiogram meant, and she somehow managed to, for the first time in my life, hide her concern.

Against all logic and all knowledge I had of the world, a world where very frequently very many things go wrong suddenly, in the Book of Laura, Laura does not have two things go very wrong on the same day. Wanting to get the most out of my morning, I booked my annual physical at my OB-GYN prior to my appointment at Asheville Head, Neck and Ear (they do not subscribe to the Oxford comma). It's not a good idea to schedule more than one body part in one day for medical examinations. My OB-GYN in West Lafayette, Indiana, had told me I would not be able to have children. In the pursuit of that ever hopeful "second opinion" I thought that Dr. Jefferies in Asheville would be superior in her skill and observation and tell me my ovaries were sparkly and smooth and fully operational. I also expected the otologist at Asheville Head, Neck and Ear to dispel my mother's hypothesis and discount her friend's stupid little machine and agree with Nanny that nothing's wrong at all and all of this is indeed a silly waste of time. I believed a doctor-day would cancel all my anxieties and fears and put everyone else's to rest as well so I could get on with my yet young life. I was meeting my ailments head-on to make them disappear. I was sure I was fine. I was thirty-two years old. Not only would I have children, I would hear every word they said. I believed that. I not only believed. I knew it. There was no room for doubt regarding any of this.

"Polycystic Ovarian Syndrome" read the pamphlet my first doctor of the day handed me, confirming the diagnosis of the other doctor and even taking it up a notch, "You won't be able to conceive, and it is even unlikely with major medical interventions." This news went against generations of women giving birth in my family. Standing up from the examining table wrapped in paper clothing, I envisioned the ancestor women all pregnant, all the way back to Nanny's Belfast and beyond that to the Border Rievers raiding spoils of other clans all along Hadrian's Wall, and far beyond that to the wilds of Britannia long before it was named Britannia. A room of suffragettes and raiders glared at me.

"When will I be a great-grandmother?" Nanny once asked me when I brought a boyfriend to meet her.

"You're great already, Nanny," I said. It would be harder to tell Nanny this news than it was to hear it myself. I had to actually pretend I had not heard it all and pull myself together for my next appointment. From Asheville Women's Medical Center, I drove to Asheville Head, Neck and Ear. The drive took ten minutes to the north end of Hendersonville Road through the pebbledash architecture of Biltmore Village from the medical mile of Ashland Avenue that leads into downtown. Ten minutes is all it took. Ten minutes to reimagine my life. Ten minutes to subtract people I had never met from a story I would never be able to tell.

"This will go much better," I assured myself and walked in through the series of glass doors.

I was the youngest person in the waiting room and found this comforting, as though my age would protect me from whatever was wrong in *their* heads, necks, and ears. I thumbed through a copy of *AARP* and reminded myself to call TIAA-CREF about the pie chart on my retirement plan. I thought I'd like to put more into real estate, less into stocks, and then something on the table caught my eye. An issue of *SEVENTEEN*, and below that, *Highlights for Children*. Within a moment of seeing the familiar primary-colored-and-white graphic and feeling the edge of a desire to do a third grade word-search, one of my former students walked into the waiting room. He was nineteen years old and had just graduated. I asked if he was there doing research for a paper for college. "No," he said, "I'm going deaf." He added, "Why are you here?" I couldn't answer.

Stretched back in the ear examining chair, Dr. Powell maneuvered the narrow tip of the otoscope around the one part of my body I'd spent the least amount of time in my life thinking about.

"Did a lot of swimming as a kid, didn't you?" he simultaneously asked and stated.

"Is that what's causing the problem?" I asked, certain he could reach for some special kind of Q-Tip and undo seventeen years of summers spent swimming in Canada's morning lakes. It would be soaked in vinegar and alcohol, like the Q-Tips my mother keeps in a shot glass at the cottage, perpetually soaking to help us prevent swimmers' ear. I thought I might have a painless case of swimmer's ear, pictured the drops on my bathroom shelf, and made a note to purchase more.

"No, it has nothing do with what's happening now." Poke, poke, poke with the otoscope. He struck the sides of my head with a tuning fork then sent me down the hall for a hearing test. There, at the end of hall from Dr. Powell's office, I met Andy the audiologist. Andy was around my age, late twenties to early thirties, with a kind face and floppy hair—an American Hugh Grant, from the *Four Weddings* days. He led me into a padded room, never an encouraging sight, but with Andy what could go wrong? Then I saw the window into a darkness. It was as though I were a contestant on the game show *Twenty-One*. He invited me to sit in a chair, then placed headphones over my ears. He attached wires to the headphones then exited, then reappeared, within seconds, in the darkness on the other side of the glass, to ask me questions just like the ones my mother's friend had. There were beeps. There were words. The words sounded defined and easy to repeat back to him. The tones were clear, and I confidently pressed the little button on the handheld device each time I heard one. When I didn't hear one, I sometimes pressed anyway. I needed a win.

Andy continues to be one of my favorite people on the planet despite the fact that, after a delightfully congenial session involving the beeps and tones and "repeat after me" games, he leveled me with the words "sensorineural hearing loss" and "listening devices." I didn't know what on earth he was talking about. Even after he explained that "listening devices" are "hearing aids" I still didn't understand what on earth he was talking about. I thought he was flirting. I expected him to leave his little dark room and come into my little dark room, punch my arm, crack up, and invite me out for a beer. It is completely fitting with my entire approach to this event that I would confuse thirty minutes in an audiometry booth with being on a date.

But there he sat on the other side of the glass, talking about these things: "Basically, you have the hearing of a seventy-five year old man . . . once we know, we can get you fitted and you'll have your listening devices by the end of the month . . . the hearing loss, if that is the only problem, is sensorineural in nature . . . it is degenerative . . . and there is no knowing how it will degenerate . . . for some it takes many years . . . for others it can be sudden and complete . . . not like vision loss . . . mild to moderate now . . . severe . . . profound . . . can wake up and hear nothing at all." It seemed that my hearing got progressively worse while he was talking to me. By the end of his explanation, I only saw his moving lips. The glass between was dark so the non-hearing person couldn't read lips, I realized. Everything was rigged against the person on my side of the booth. And the window did not lower so Andy could not reach across and take my hand and assure me everything was going to be alright. Instead it was like listening to a flight attendant rattle off the crash instructions . . . Place the oxygen on yourself first and then your child. . . ." A calm, unthreatening voice saying dire, threatening things. "You have the hearing of a seventy-five-year-old man."

And then the strange assurance lifted its head in the form of his words, "At this time, we aren't absolutely positive." And in that moment, through the glass darkly, I saw what I thought was a sheen of hope in Andy's eyes. Something positive. Some accusation against the certainty of all the beeps, tones, and words, against the computer, darkness and cold glass, against science itself. Maybe all of this was wrong. I reached for the Flonase in my purse.

"It could be Lupus or a brain tumor." The glass darkened further. "We'll have to draw some blood."

With a cotton ball and a blue strip of surgical tape strapped to my inner-elbow, I returned to Christ School to teach the boys *Beowulf* for the last period of class. Late August shadows covered us as we walked through the woods.

"Stay in the path, boys!" I shouted as poison ivy slouched toward the cuffs of their khakis. I always taught *Beowulf* in the woods, and today I needed to be in the woods more than anything. I had started out, during my first year at Christ School, in the classroom, but hearing the boys read from their desks about battle and heroism and the slaying of monsters and dragons made such little sense. They comprised the pantheon of learning-style difference poster-boys. They needed to be outside. Since that first fall, I had acquired a closet-full of faux fur and plastic medieval weaponry that could do in a pinch when we reached Macbeth a few weeks later. We moved quickly through the evolution of British literature. A mere wink and we'd go from Anglo-Saxon warriors to Chivalric knights to lacy-frilled cavaliers. Through poems and plays and stories we rode the arc of the centuries it takes to try to civilize men. I loved the *Beowulf* part of the year. Standing in a meadow near the old stone ruins of a cottage on a lower field, I handed out the weapons and the boys cloaked themselves in fake fur and started to fight while Parker Crecenzo held a video camera and filmed. Shane McEnany coached the fighting pairs in stage combat because he had taken a course at camp. Calvin Blake banged a drum he had bought on a Saturday excursion into downtown Asheville where drums are for sale in about ten small shops. Old drums. When Calvin brought it to class, he was so excited to have something to contribute to the battle scenes, I completely bought into the idea that of course all Anglo-Saxon battles were fought to a beat. While they fought around him, Dave Porter read from the text on whatever page we were on:

> I knew him of yore in his youthful days;
> his aged father was Ecgtheow named,
> to whom, at home, gave Hrethel the Geat
> his only daughter. Their offspring bold
> fares hither to seek the steadfast friend.

It was not absolutely necessary to have men fighting behind Hrothgar as he tells his men about the great warrior to the north, but we were all in this for drama. Weapons flew through the air, crashed in negative space. Parker called, "Cut and print." There'd be no printing. None of us knew anything about editing.

We moved up the meadow toward the lake to film Grendel and his mom. All the boys wanted to be play Grendel's mom, but the role went to Matt Housely because he could make the most frightening noises, ungodly noises, which is what the whole monk-revised script calls for. Our Beowulf was played by Sam from the spectrum because he thrived with scripted speech. The other boys cheered him as Sam wielded his mighty sword, Hrunting, above the water of the dark lake where dwelled Matt Housely's terrifying "sea-witch."

As they cheered and roared, as Beowulf explains to a loving BFF Wiglaf, played by Alex Finley, that he will not be able to use his usual sword under the water, I lost myself in their enthusiasm for the project if not for the literature. Where we were was so quiet and removed from the usual busyness of campus. Here, we could not hear a bell ring or a car engine, and no one could hear the death shriek of Grendel's mother. The century-old, five-thousand-acre wooded campus allowed these timeless spaces. Parker filmed Sam and Matt fighting in the shallows. It was the last period of the day, so the boys insisted it did not matter if they got wet and muddy. I believed them and frankly did not care. To film the underwater battle, the two boys submerged, creating turbulence on the surface, that Parker insisted he could loop to make it look like a much longer battle once filming completed. A bell did ring through the trees, and the boys heard it. With battle axes slung over their shoulders and fake fur soaked from bored off-camera boys wearing it into the water to cool off, we returned along the path. We passed the headmaster's house, passed the old log cabin a former headmaster owned but seldom visited, and upon arriving at the front steps of Wetmore Hall, were greeted by the headmaster himself and the bishop of the Diocese of North Carolina.

"Good afternoon, sir," my ragged and embattled boys said politely as they passed.

"Good afternoon," said Father Ingersoll and the bishop.

"We're reading *Beowulf*, sir." I said as the boys filed through the double glass doors with their weapons, which they put away neatly in the closet in my classroom, returning to their preppy tidy selves, if you don't count the soaking wet boys or the mud and face paint.

"See you tomorrow, Ms. Hope."

When they left the room, I noticed that the little cotton ball and tape were still on the inside of my elbow. Actually, I noticed I had forgotten about it for the time we had been roaming and waging battle in the forest. It wasn't a normal kind of forgetting. I had dissociated entirely. I pulled at the blue tape and stared at the red blood on the cotton. For all the bloodshed in *Beowulf*, it was this that terrified me. I put my head down on my desk and cried.

I stared at the map of the human ear outside my audiologist's office. The map was three feet wide and two feet tall and provided detailed anatomy of ear canals and ear bones. After three months of wearing listening devices, I had completed a required check-in. There are three parts to this check-in. The first is the geographical, the actual act of getting to and arriving at the Asheville head, neck, and ear place and sitting in the waiting room. The second is the technical, which involves going back into the black box of silence and being spoken to through a wall of darkened glass. The third is the adjustment of the devices.

In the audiometry booth, a new audiologist (Andy had quit to pursue his dream of being a goat-farmer, no kidding), named Beth connected my devices with wires to her computer and asked me what levels she needed to change. We went through the test, with the syllables and the beeps, and the little button to press. I was now recalling the opening credits of *The Bionic Woman*. I had never understood what Jamie Somers was doing with the headphones and why she crushed a tennis ball after. Where was my tennis ball? After the tests, we left the room of silence and went to her office. The office was small and quiet, unlike any of the settings in which I wore hearing aids. She was very cheerful and optimistic about everything. I saw on the certificate behind her that she had only had her degree for six months. To help her feel useful and accomplished I asked to make a few random adjustments and assured, "Oh yes, that's much better." I had no idea what the world sounded like and shouldn't sound like. From what I'd seen and heard of it in the past three months nothing in Beth's little office could possibly improve matters. I did not like Beth. Beth could ask me a million questions and none of them would be the right ones because I felt none of them had anything to do with the actual internal experience of going deaf. It was not about noise or directional microphones or music settings or t-coils and loops, words that I really didn't understand and had no way of knowing of evaluating or even wanting them. Losing hearing was about losing people and losing my sense of my place in the world. Beth was a fixer. She needed to feel that hearing aids fixed deafness. We had just participated in a forced tableau wherein science and silence had pretended to have a conversation, and we had pretended that we had been successful.

There is no success in the first year of diagnosis of anything. Vials can fill up with blood. Little lights can flare and fade in response to responses. Everything, though, is wobbly. The new information that life will not be the same takes some time to find its way. Its way in what exactly? What exactly does it mean to *go deaf?* In my case, deafness was a whole story of its own. It had a history, and that history had characters: people who had lived it out, people like Beethoven and Helen Keller (though not the real one but the Melissa Gilbert covered in sand one), people like the baseball team that invented hand-signs because one of the players was deaf. Deafness had a mythos that dwelled as far from my own as the idea of my ever becoming a racecar driver. It was something I had never thought about. Standing and looking at the three-foot long and two-foot tall poster of the interior architecture of the human ear, I recognized what had gone wrong in Beth's quiet little office.

Audiology and the poster and even the hearing aids were all about the *logos* of hearing loss. They had it all measured, quantified on my audiogram with my cookie-bite hearing loss right across the speech banana. They had *hearing* completely figured out. What they did not know how to talk about was the *loss.* And that is what every diagnosis is really about: what you are about to lose, what you are in the process of losing, what other people will lose as whatever condition you have proceeds. And also—and this is powerful—what you will gain.

I was too early in this process to have my own story of deafness, my own mythos. So, standing in front of the poster, I found myself making up a story from the names of the parts of the ear. There were semicircular canals, a bony labyrinth, a cochlea that looked as much as it sounded like a seashell. There were tympanic membranes—the drums! And there was even something called the auricle. I could see the mythic quest developing before my eyes as young cochlea entered the canals and made her way through the bony labyrinth. She had to quietly creep past the tympanic membrane lest the evil stapes be alerted to her presence and attack her with their malleus's. If she was successful, and it was a very big *if,* she could secure the auricle and save all the kingdom of incus.

"Can I help you with anything?" Beth asked as she emerged from her office in her scrub suit. It made no sense that the audiologists wore scrub suits that lent themselves to an increased anxiety factor as though at any moment they could become surgeons.

How could I answer her without undoing all the glamor of what we had created in her office, the illusion that she had done her job just fine and my hearing aids were now perfectly attuned to my world and my needs? I was so tempted to explain to her that my heart was broken in the presence of cold science, that I felt that what was really going on had absolutely nothing to do with the little bobbins in my ear holes. It was something of the soul I felt had been damaged in all of this, that I didn't know where I belonged anymore or if I belonged in the world at all. Beth needed to believe that the degree on her wall stood for an ability to help people with hearing loss. I so wanted to believe in that as well, but Cochlea had a long way to go to safely traverse the bony labyrinth. Not many had been successful in the past. The ones who failed were never heard from again. A sad story was telling itself in my imagination.

"No, I'm good," I said to Beth, And Beth walked on. I stayed longer to study the map of the human ear. I was further deluding myself that the answers lay in knowledge, in awareness of all of the parts. I recalled my grandfather dismantling and reassembling an old pocket watch over a black velvet cloth all the parts shimmered against. When he was finished he held the timepiece between two pressed hands then held it close to his ear and announced it was working.

"But, Poppee, there are two pieces still on the velvet."

"They were what was wrong."

What I was looking at the posters for was something wrong. And I needed something very specific that was wrong—dying little furry nerves simply were not enough.

My encounters with the medical side of deafness had so far always left me feeling isolated. Violently pushed aside, even if the conversation was about my own ears. This map I stood before, if it were posted on the wall vertically instead of horizontally, would be the length of my torso. That is how conversations with audiologists made me feel: like I was a giant ear with legs.

Back when I taught on the Olympic Peninsula I read a *TIME* magazine article about how a group of scientists had successfully grown an adult-sized human ear on an otherwise small white mouse. With its own tiny pink ears and its tiny pink eyes and tail, the inset photograph featured the anomalous evidence: a mouse with an enormous human ear on its back. An excellent ear by all counts if you overlook the fact that it's grown on the back of a mouse inside the mouse's skin and liberation of this ear from this mouse will cost that mouse its life. In the photograph, the mouse is clearly alive and just terrified (when do mice not look terrified?) about this whole situation. Of course, the ear was a mere likeness of an ear. It would befit someone whose actual ear had been terribly damaged in an act of war, a factory accident, or a fire. This is the replacement ear for someone without one. It could help Vincent Van Gogh. It couldn't, though, replace my ear. My ears are great. They stick out just the right amount. They didn't always. When I was ten I used my ears to pin my hair back like Lori Partridge of *The Partridge Fami-*

ly, only my hair was much thicker than Lori Partridge's. When my family traveled that summer in Europe, border agents would flip through the four passports my father handed them then actually laugh or crack a smile and look up when they got to mine, to prove to themselves that someone had ears like mine. From that era, I still cringe at the mention of Dumbo the Elephant, taking it personally. But my ears have flattened back now. As for that mouse, though, I could relate now more to that mouse as a map of my hearing loss than to the actual map in front of me.

That mouse understood what it's like to have an appendage that doesn't make sense and that forms rather a weight upon one's being and feels exaggerated in size, disproportionate to the actuality of one's self. When people viewed that photograph in *TIME* all those years ago, no one was looking at little laboratory mouse number 67 billion 987 thousand 453. No. They were looking at the ear growing out of its back. But the mouse itself was a miracle enough by many counts. I, too, had been rather okay and my own little miracle just moving along in the world prior to this hearing loss event. I had been quite fine. Now, everything was about these ears. They were always what I thought about. They had nothing to do with what I saw when I looked in the mirror because I had these special invisible hearing aids from Re-Sound, a name suggesting the first Sound had failed, I'd like to point out. I had been ReSounded, remade in the image of the little mouse nervously attached to an artificial sonic device. Terrified. Prey not of hawks and eagles but of beeps and tones and wires affixed to my devices. I was a little laboratory mouse in my own right, using the first-generation of the latest Completely-in-the-Canal listening devices. The information I had given to Beth was now being graphed and fed into the engineering data at ReSound. ReSound would then ReSound itself and come up with another generation of artificial ears on the forms of little brightly colored almonds. NASA would soon learn about me. And still, I'd be the jittery little mouse named Cochlea making my way through the maze of sound, the bony labyrinth.

Once I had found a metaphor and a story and an analogy, I felt I could actually turn away from the giant map of the human ear and return home. I had solved something. I even felt I had figured out the first turn of the maze. I even had a little inkling of what the little piece of cheese might be at the end of it all. It would not be having my hearing restored. That was impossible. The little piece of cheese would be being alright without being able to hear. The maze was long. I understood that. It might even be interminable. And that did not matter. I was in it, and it was my new life's path to navigate it as well as I could. I exited into the waiting area where children and people my age and people three times my age waited in a large room for their name to be called, which many of them wouldn't even hear. That was how insane this realm of audiology was. Everyone should be given one of those vibrating discs they give you when you're waiting for a table in a restaurant. Otherwise, everyone just sits in a state of stress, unsure what sound the receptionist will make next.

My hearing aids lie nestled in a blue ceramic tea cup with a little strainer built in and a lid. The devices go into the strainer, and the lid quietly shuts them in. I painted a little scene of an Italian villa on the side of the cup at the little paint-your-own-pottery shops in downtown Asheville. It wasn't my intention to make a special place for my hearing aids, but I like this. It is ceremonial and beautiful, and I like to treat the devices with such reverence now as befits a special vessel. I've come to love them as I've come to love my deafness.

I think back to the year of diagnosis, 2001, a year in which I traveled to England, Puerto Rico, and China, all after 9-11, had three love affairs, and finished the earth's journey around the sun pregnant (no medical interventions required) with a girl who is now fifteen. I see so clearly now the darkness of the audiometry booth and the disconnected manner of my diagnosis—how the very moment of my diagnosis shaped that early narrative. Deafness has a terribly cold and disconnected feeling to it in a culture that destroys silence. Those two qualities dominated my instant of being told. But it is not cold and disconnected at all. I recognize the moment at the poster as the beginning of my living into deafness. Hardly a quick fix, finding a mythos in diagnosis is a lifelong project. It is an opening to a story but not the story itself. Joseph Campbell writes of poets who "possess the courage to follow the echoes of the eloquence within." I was a poet before deafness, and I am more of one as the "cookie-bite" of the audiogram has descended far below the "speech banana." Finding meaning in diagnosis requires poetry, requires metaphor, requires that we bridge the body to the whole wide world with words, requires story. Otherwise it is what is cold and disconnected and removes us from life.

After I mused on the mouse with the ear on its back, I started to search for other stories that would help me tell my own. It was not a process that came consciously. To access meaning in deafness, I had to sit and write. To be honest, I did not write immediately. I was pregnant against all odds and became a single mother as rapidly as I became a mother at all. I wrote when my daughter was three and old enough to occupy herself with paints and crayons, and I could exhale a bit. The first essay was one about my grandfather who was deaf but who never presented himself as disabled. I had to take ownership of disability for both of us. He also was an English teacher, though, so I found I wove poetry into speaking of deafness, and this reframed the disability with a new dimension. I further explored that dimension with an essay in which I meditated on the way "silence" and "deafness" and "hearing" are used in sacred texts and connected these to images I saw in the dome of St. Paul's that first wild year of diagnosis: images of the prophets and apostles in various stages of "hearing God" and writing down God's words. After that I rather figured out the game: while writing did not cure deafness, it moved me into it and helped me find what it meant. It was not a hollow silence at all but a rich labyrinth of echoes of a world I no longer hear without the assistance of technology. In some odd way, except for hearing my friends, students, and family, I honestly do not need to hear it anymore. By moving it into words, I moved the world into me.

The process was not at all somber or reverent. One night, I was up writing and turned on the TV to take a little break. On the screen, in that hopeful scene in *2001: A Space Odyssey*, Poole and Bowman are huddled in the little escape pod plotting to disconnect the psychotic computer, Hal, before Hal kills them off. They've turned off the "com." They think they are being clever and silent. Then Bowman gets out and Hal sends Poole hurtling out into space with no means of ever getting back, and the audience watches Poole just drift off, terrifyingly alone into the soundlessness of space. My first thought was to identify with Poole.

"That's like going deaf," I said to myself, eager to begin another essay mourning my loss of hearing.

The red-light eye of Hal dominates the screen after Bowman asks, "We had the com turned off, Hal. How did you know?"

"I can read lips, Dave."

And I thought to myself, "Hmm. And so is *that*."

My daughter is the child of a deaf mother.

"Put your squishy earrings in," she used to say when she noticed I was not lipreading well.

"I don't think you heard me," she would say when I said no to a request for a popsicle.

Deafness is part of our story as neither aid nor detriment. It's a benefit when she has friends over and can laugh with them all night without having to be quiet. It's a pain when we go to a movie where the closed caption devices aren't functioning well. On the whole, it has taught her patience and humor. On the whole, it has taught me that love has nothing to do with ability or the five senses. The most important moments between us, as anyone knows, are when nothing is spoken at all and she just knows I am there for her. We sign our own sign language which we have cooked up together. She knows how to crack me up from across the room with a funny song we composed one summer years ago involving a little piece of poop floating in a public pool. I never yelled at her while she was growing up and instead signed, "Put that down right now. I love you," when she nabbed a candy bar in line at the grocery store. She grew up peacefully possibly because of the lack of the stress of yelling. She also signed her first sentence long before her first spoken words. She signed "done" at nine months and applied it to everything from being finished eating to telling the doctor about to give her a shot, "you're done." It's not the American Sign Language (ASL) that would survive in the real world, but it binds us in our own.

I wear Phonak hearing aids now. I wear Phonak completely behind the ear (BTE) that are the color of "Merlot" to match my lipstick because I actually want people to know I am deaf and they need to step up the conversation skills and Look At Me. I switched to Phonak because they had a team in the Tour de France, and I developed a crush on the whole lot of them cruising along the Mediterranean in tight Phonak jerseys. I was still searching for real-world metaphors for deafness, and a whole team of fit people on bikes in France worked for me. People ask me if I'll get cochlear implants. They ask, I think, because they are saddened by my deafness. They want to see me "whole" or fixed. It is odd that the solution that comes to mind involves drilling a hole in my head and severing what living nerves I have left so I can wear hearing aids just like I do now. I smile at them and assure them that my hearing aids will work very well for a very long time, taking almost nothing and amplifying it pretty much to the level at which they hear. I then tell them, "And I can take them out." And they get it. This double world of loud and quiet, a symphony in my head. There is only one thing I mourn, something no device can fix, just so no one thinks not everything is perfect now.

Every summer I still return to the Northwoods of Ontario. My daughter and I make the trip up the Appalachians then across the Niagara and the Ontario Prairie. We reach the rocky shores of Georgian Bay where my grandmother did eventually get to hold her great-grand-daughter and where the 4.4-billion-year-old rocks support our little cottage and lead us down into the blue water. I remove my hearing aids and place them in a little travel case beside my bed. I then paddle out in a canoe just as I did all those mornings in childhood. And I wait. I wait for it. I wait for that beautiful call that soars upon the ancient air but that is threatened now and heard less often even by those who are not deaf. I call out. I call out again, and I hope, I hope it hears me.

Chapter Seven

Living with Interstitial Cystitis

An Autoethnography of Developing and Coping with a Chronic Condition

Jessica M. W. Kratzer

I stood looking at myself in the bathroom mirror wondering what was happening to me. My body has been through so much these past eight months and now this. I wasn't sure how much more I could handle. I was caring for an infant and toddler so I was tired. I was living in a state where I had no family support other than my husband. I stared at myself thinking how my body could heal when more problems were arising. I was recovering from childbirth, dealing with a postpartum physical problem that required physical therapy, and now I was urinating blood. It was all too much.

    The purpose of this chapter is to share my experiences with the onset of a chronic condition in my thirties. As you follow this story, you will be shown aspects of my life that were challenging and painful, both physically and emotionally. However, please remember that this is only one aspect of my life. There were many good and happy things happening during this time, but my condition, interstitial cystitis (IC) was also part of it all. IC was in the background all of the time and in the forefront often, but I still had many wonderful aspects of my life that have made the struggle bearable. I will invite you to walk through my journey by informing you of my health history, the onset of my condition, the impact it had on me, and eventually learning to cope with it. Before reading my story, it is important to understand my condition.

    "Interstitial Cystitis (IC) is a relatively rare, painful bladder condition, characterized by urinary urgency, frequency, and lower abdominal pain" (Webster, 1996, p. 197). Webster (1996) states that urinary urgency can be especially difficult because the body no longer uses normal signals to indicate a full bladder; instead the bladder spasms. These spasms may radiate causing pain in the lower back or abdomen. The abdomen pain can range from a heavy pain to a sharp, needle-like pain. Urgency of urination can be as frequent as every fifteen minutes, which can be quite distressing for daytime functioning and can disrupt regular sleep patterns. IC is commonly treated with installations of medications released directly into the bladder via a catheter. My experience with IC includes all of the descriptors above. When my bladder gets inflamed, I have lower abdomen pain that radiates harshly if someone bumps my stomach. I have to urinate often, which means I have to leave the classes I am teaching or the meetings I am in to use the restroom. I also wake up during the night often and have installations of medications to calm my bladder. These are the symptoms that affect my body, and they are direct and generally easy to understand. However, IC is much more than a set of symptoms; it is a way of life. I will take you on my autoethnographic journey with IC so that you can understand how the onset of this chronic condition has affected me in ongoing and life-altering ways.

AUTOETHNOGRAPHY AND THE IMPORTANCE OF SHARING PERSONAL EXPERIENCES

Autoethnography is a form of qualitative inquiry that systematically describes and analyzes a person's first-hand experiences and connects those experiences to social and cultural contexts (Ettorre, 2016). Specifically, it focuses on the product of the experience and the process of the inquiry (Ellis, 2004). This means that the story of how you got to where you are, what happened, and how it happened are just as important as what you learned at the conclusion. Autoethnography is usually written in first-person, which is why I am writing this chapter as if I am talking to you. I want you to feel as if you are a fly on the wall of my life. Scholars use a variety of forms that may include short stories, novels, fiction, scripts, social science prose, etc. (Ellis, Adams, & Bochner, 2011; Ellis, 2004). I will use a personal narrative to share my experiences. Using a layered account (Ronai, 1992), I share my experiences through story-telling, dialogue, emotions, and academic prose to give you a clear understanding of my story and how it relates to health communication.

I use autoethnography to tell a health narrative, which is a way for patients to make sense of their illness (Babrow, Kline, & Rawlins, 2005). According to Spieldenner (2014), "These narratives often present with culturally embedded symbols that reveal personal and social beliefs about sickness" (p. 14). Health narratives are used to make meaning of an individual's illness in terms of the context of the illness, the time it takes to deal with the illness, and their attempts to cope with it (Babrow et al., 2005). While there are many benefits of health narratives, they can also be problematic because storytellers can use symbols in error or they may have difficulty telling their stories (Harter, Japp, & Beck, 2005). Additionally, their perspective may be different from others dealing with the same illness or others involved in the patient's health experiences. For instance, "Patient-provider relations unfold as the coconstruction of narrative knowledge" (Harter & Bochner, 2009). This means that my doctors and nurses co-created a narrative of information sharing with me. However, the stories you will read in this chapter are only from my perspective and do not include the involvement of my healthcare providers, whose memories and perspectives likey differ from mine.

When learning about medical problems, we expect doctors, nurses, and other healthcare practitioners to provide us with the best information possible. While this is an expectation that we should have as patients, it should not discount the experiences of the people who have been directly affected by illness, disability, and other medical problems (Richards, 2008). Sharing my experiences with chronic illness as a health narrative is valid because I have lived it and can tell you what it feels like rather than what it looks like. According to Richards (2008),

> People living with disabilities or illnesses are seen as objects of study and not as agents of study. There seems to be an underlying assumption that such people need to be talked about, but should themselves remain silent as if they do not have anything useful to contribute. They are also frequently the recipients of other people's expertise, not the contributors. (p. 1719)

You can look up interstitial cystitis online or ask a doctor about it, but reading about my personal account can give you further insight into how one person lives with this condition. Therefore, a combination of resources is most helpful in understanding a medical condition.

Throughout the chapter, you will observe how I discovered my condition, how I coped with it over the past several years, and how I learned to embrace it as part of my life. According to Bochner and Ellis (2006), autoethnography also allows readers to witness the author "learning how to live, struggling to make sense of their lives and their losses, healing their wounds, trying to move on from and survive the unnerving blows of fate to which all of us are vulnerable" (p. 118). Even more powerful for me as the writer, is that I can understand the process of gaining control of my body by sharing my experiences with you. Therefore, this chapter has been a learning experience for me as I have written it. I hope it will be educational for you as well.

Additionally, this chapter focuses on my health, which is private information. "In the context of illness, this [autoethnography] can offer a therapeutic experience for the author even if it sometimes requires uncomfortable personal disclosure" (Withnall, 2017). This means that I will share very personal and private information about my life and my body with you. This is a vulnerable position to be in both because I am telling you intimate aspects of myself but also because I risk humiliation (Jago, 2002) and being viewed as defective (Richards, 2008). I am willing to share my story to help myself cope, and to help you have a better understanding of how some people may deal with a chronic condition. The following autoethnographic essay is my attempt to work through my process of coping with interstitial cystitis, and I am happy, yet nervous, to share it with you.

MY HEALTH

I was healthy my entire life with no notable problems outside normal illnesses until my husband and I tried to conceive a baby. At age thirty, I was found to have endometriosis, which affected my ability to get pregnant. Endometriosis is an often-painful disorder where the tissue that lines the inside of the uterus grows outside of the uterus. It can grow on the ovaries, fallopian tubes, tissues lining the pelvis, and other organs (e.g., bladder). Endometriosis cannot leave the body naturally, so it continues to grow and creates scar tissue that causes pain and fertility problems (Mayo Clinic, 2018a). At age thirty-one, a doctor surgically removed most of the endometriosis, and I got pregnant a month later. Two years after that we conceived another baby without fertility assistance. Three weeks after my second child was born, I discovered that I had a prolapsed organ. A pelvic organ prolapse is when the ligaments and muscles that support a woman's pelvic organs is weakened and the organs drop lower in the pelvis, which creates a budge, or prolapse, in the vagina (Mayo Clinic, 2018b). Over the next few months, I was found to have three prolapses (bladder, uterus, and rectum). I saw three physical therapists over the next few years, which is an entirely different story (literally, I already wrote it). During the same time that I was discovering my prolapses and trying to figure out how to cope with them, I discovered another condition.

THE INTRODUCTION OF INTERSTITIAL CYSTITIS

I was certain that I had a urinary tract infection or maybe a bladder infection. Why else would there be blood in my urine? My primary physician tested me and found that I had neither. After a round of antibiotics did not improve my condition, I went to see a urologist. The urology nurse practitioner, Eve, tested my urine and found a lot of blood in it. She scheduled me to have an exploratory surgery where the urologist sent a camera through my urethra and into my bladder to see what was going on. When I came out of the anesthesia, the urologist told me that the lining of my bladder was very angry, irritated, and cracked. The cracking of my bladder's lining was bleeding, accounting for the blood in my urine. He said that I had something called interstitial cystitis. He reviewed what this condition was, but I do not remember much because I was in a fog from the anesthesia. This was the only time I ever spoke directly with the urologist. All my visits for the next two years were with the nurse practitioner or a registered nurse. At my follow-up appointment, Eve, the nurse practitioner at the urology office, explained what my condition was and what I could expect to experience.

"You have interstitial cystitis, which is a condition that is caused by a trauma to the abdomen, usually from a car accident or something similar. Your trauma was giving birth to your son, who was a very large baby. The use of forceps could have added to the trauma. The lining of your bladder can no longer expand as much as it used to without cracking and bleeding. The urgency you feel to urinate often is also from IC because your bladder can no longer hold as much urine."

"Ok, what needs to be done to fix this?" I asked, completely overwhelmed yet under the impression that IC was, in fact, fixable. I had never had any form of illness in my life that did not have a remedy.

"There's nothing you can do to get rid of IC. You will have it for the rest of your life," Eve said, trying to be as understanding as possible. My head is swimming. Nothing had prepared me for this moment, a moment that felt like it would never end. I could not believe that I would have this forever. The pain would continue. I never thought I would have a condition that would affect me forever with absolutely no cure. I tried not to cry but was unsuccessful.

She looked at me sympathetically and continued, "But, we can help you manage it. We can give you a treatment where I use a catheter to insert medication directly into your bladder that will calm it down and reduce the bleeding and pain."

"How often do I need to have these treatments?" I asked, wiping my eyes.

"It depends on how long they will work for you. I will give you a treatment today and then you can make an appointment when your bladder starts to hurt. We can usually get you in the same day or the next. Let's start with a treatment today and see how you feel."

Eve gave me a treatment that day. She inserted a very small catheter meant for babies because she said it should cause less discomfort. (Although I had a regular catheter once before, I did not remember what having a catheter felt like.) In that moment, it felt like the baby catheter was scraping my urethra all the way up. I could not imagine what a regular catheter would feel like . . . it must be much worse. In less than three weeks, the pain was back. I started going to the urology office every three weeks for over a year. The second year of having IC I went to the office for treatments every five weeks. This affected so many aspects of my life including leaving work early for treatments, coordinating schedules with my husband, knowing where the restroom was located every place I went, my teaching arrangements, my lack of privacy, and anxiety about pain. The continued invasion of, and lack of control over my body overwhelmed and exhausted me.

I had to keep the medicine in my bladder for one hour before urinating. This sounds like a simple task, but it was very difficult for two reasons. First, my bladder was already irritated. So, I had the urgency to urinate often. Not going to the restroom when my bladder was full of medication was very difficult. Second, my pelvic floor muscles were weak. I had even less muscle control after a treatment. This meant that I would leak the medication very easily. I had to be careful lifting things, bending over, and making any quick movements for a full hour. This was very difficult because I was toting around a toddler and a baby. My husband could sometimes get home in time to keep the kids while I had a treatment, but the urology office closed at 4:30 pm and he worked forty-five minutes away. More times than not I had to take my kids with me. While I received treatment, they would sit in the stroller next to the doctor's table I was lying on, eating their snacks. It was important for me to stay lying down for a few minutes after the treatment to help my body settle and hold in the medicine. Then I would have to take the kids back to the van, load them into car seats, and pack up my huge double stroller. These activities created more pain in my bladder and made it difficult to avoid leaking the medication immediately following a treatment.

IC RULING MY LIFE

Living with interstitial cystitis was very stressful. This was my life. While it was not terminal, and the pain was not completely debilitating (thanks to the medication), and I knew that many people had conditions much worse than mine, it still affected my body and mind negatively. IC was constantly at the forefront of my thoughts. When would it start to hurt? Would it be on a weekend when I could not get a treatment? What if I went out of town and the pain started? I knew where every restroom was every time I went anywhere. Festivals and other large public gatherings made me nervous (I avoided these as much as I could). Where is the restroom? How long are the lines? How far away am I willing to be from a restroom? Long car rides had me in knots and always worried about traffic or when we would stop. On a vacation to visit my brother, my biggest concern was going to the beach. I needed to be near a restroom, so my brother led us to a place on the beach that had public facilities. In addition to having the urgency, it was important that I not wait too long to go to the restroom or it would be difficult for me to walk. In those moments, every single step felt like my bladder was daring me to take one hard step or two rushed steps that would open the gates and I would pee everywhere. Fortunately, my bladder never won that dare but it got close several times.

IC also affected my work life. On several occasions, I had to leave the class I was teaching to urinate because I could not hold it any longer. The worst was when I had to leave a class while a guest speaker was presenting. I requested that I teach near a restroom after that embarrassing incident. I taught all over campus and some classrooms were far away from the restrooms, or so it seemed to me, and I was too afraid to be that far from relief. Fortunately, the chair of my department accommodated my needs. According to McGonagle and Adams-Farrell (2013), perceptions of identity threats in the workplace can be stressful for people with chronic illness. I did not want to tell my supervisor about my condition but I had to. Interstitial cystitis threatened my identity as a full-functioning, healthy, independent employee. It was very private information to share.

In May 2016, I had my last treatment with Eve. I was moving to a different state that week and needed to find a new urologist right away. I was afraid to find a new doctor because I thought that the treatment I was getting with Eve was the best there was. Moving and leaving Eve ended up being so much better for my situation. Leaving was the start of gaining more control over my body and my life.

HOPE ON THE HORIZON

Two weeks later I was sitting on a paper covered table waiting to meet my new doctor. Waiting to see if he would want to make changes to my treatment, waiting to see if I would like him. Waiting to see if he would value my experiences and give me the medication I needed to relieve my pain. It was all very overwhelming; my anxiety and uncertainty were taking over my entire thought process. Waiting. The door opened and in walked a short Caucasian man with a white mustache and white hair. He was wearing dark slacks, a collared white shirt, tie, and physician's jacket.

"Hello, Jessica. I am Dr. Adams. What can I do for you today?" he asked, in a very soft, kind voice.

"Hi, Dr. Adams. Well, I have just moved here from Tennessee and I need a new urologist to give me treatments for my interstitial cystitis. I brought the files from my previous physician with me, so you have the information regarding what has been going on over the past two years. I currently get a treatment every five weeks."

"I read your information and I have a few options for you. First, let me say that each doctor has their own preferences on the types of medications used to manage IC. I like to call them cocktails. Your previous physician used a cocktail that contained a few different medications. Some of which I don't have but can order them. One medication in their cocktail is not one I can send home with you because it can only be opened right before use. I cannot measure it out to send it home since it has such a short shelf life," he explained. Home? Why would he send it home with me? I continued to listen. "I prefer to use one medication called Marcaine. I use 30 milliliters and have you keep it in your bladder for thirty minutes."

"I've always had to keep my previous medications in for at least an hour," I said.

"You only need to keep this in for thirty minutes. It doesn't do any extra good if you keep it in longer. The benefit of using this medication is that I can teach you how to catheterize yourself and you can take it home with you. This will greatly reduce the amount of in-office visits you have to make and will likely reduce the amount of medication you use. Research has shown that when we give the patient the power to administer their own medication, they tend to use it much less for a few reasons. First, they do not feel the need to rush to the office to get a treatment before the weekend or leaving town. Second, they are more willing to monitor the way their bladder feels to see if it will calm down in a day or two because they can administer the medication if the irritation continues. Giving yourself the treatment gives you a great deal of freedom because you can take it anywhere you go, and you don't have to worry about scheduling a visit and being in pain longer. Would you like to consider that option?"

"Ummm, wow, I wasn't expecting that. No one has ever mentioned that I could do this myself. I, I can't believe this. Yes, I mean, I would love to do this on my own. Thank you, so much. I really just can't believe this," I said, stunned.

"Ok," he said. "Let me give you a treatment now to see if the Marcaine works for you. I'll have you come back in a month and we'll revisit the medication. If it works for you then I'll teach you how to do this yourself, and we'll send you home with all the supplies you need. How does that sound?"

"That sounds perfect," I said, still quite stunned. I could not believe that I could take care of myself without being shackled to the doctor's office. I had very low expectations for this doctor's visit and I thought someone new would try to control my body in different ways than I was accustomed to from Eve's office. Change scared me, so I wanted either the same care I received with Eve or something better, but I was not expecting something better. However, I got something better, so much better. The control over my own body, the gaining of privacy, and the hope that I would be freer to live my life and take care of myself was better than I ever thought was possible. After this, my life changed again, for the better.

Good news: The Marcaine worked for me! Dr. Adams taught me how to catheterize myself. Since then, I have only needed treatments about every six months. Additionally, he had me use adult catheters, which are far less painful than the baby ones used at my previous physician's office. Less pain when administering the medication was a relief. Catheterizing myself was very scary and overwhelming at first. Honestly, I was terrified. Dr. Adams showed me how easy it is, with some help from my husband. The first time I did it, I was shaking, but it worked. Catheterizing myself was so much easier than I thought it would be.

The process of getting the power to take care of my body on my own terms has changed everything. I no longer have the lingering fear that I might be in pain over a weekend or before a trip if I do not get a treatment at the doctor's office. I am no longer shackled to the doctor's office with constant visits. No one else is invading my body and causing me pain. My body is mine now and no longer belongs to someone else, a freedom I took for granted before the diagnosis. Upon diagnosis, I had to let someone else invade my body and cause me pain to get relief from pain. That slowly chipped away at my self-worth. Gaining control has given me the opportunity to learn more about myself as a person, advocate for my own health moving forward, and know my body better.

I have allowed myself to listen to my body more carefully. Sometimes my bladder hurts for reasons that do not equate to the need for a treatment. I now know that sometimes it hurts because I need to drink more water, or I am constipated and the pressure irritates my bladder. The constipation revelation took a long time to figure out. Once I did, I have been able to manage my bowels to keep my bladder happy. I also know that my abdomen is very sensitive. I cannot roughhouse with my kids in the same way my husband can because kicks and pounces hurt my bladder. Not enough to need a treatment, but it is much more sensitive. I am aware of my bladder often. I still want to know where the restroom is located most places I go, just in case. However, I no longer leak and my capacity for holding urine has increased so I do not have to go as often. I can sleep through the night without getting up to go to the restroom. A full night of sleep on a regular basis has been helpful for my body and my mental well-being.

It has been important for me to maintain a sense of self as a person with a chronic condition. I lost that sense by feeling weighed down with doctor's appointments, by knowing that pain could creep up at any time and I had no way of helping myself without getting medication at the doctor's office, and knowing that pain was going to occur when getting the treatment I needed. This weight made me feel like a slave to my condition. I was not managing interstitial cystitis; IC was running my life. While Eve, the nurse I saw regularly, had my best intentions in mind (and I truly think she did), I had no agency over my body. That affected my overall sense of self, or lack thereof.

According to Holman and Lorig (2000), a patient's self-management of their condition is enhanced when they are educated about "continuous use of medication, behavior change, pain control, adjusting to social and workplace dislocations, coping with emotional reactions, learning to interpret changes in the disease and its consequences, and use of medical and community resources" (p. 527). Additionally, and very true to my experience, educated patients experience reduced symptoms, improvement in physical activity, and a significant reduction in the need for medical treatment (Holman & Lorig, 2000). Dr. Adams educated me. That education got me on the path of improving my life and learning to cope with IC.

LIVING IN HARMONY WITH INTERSTITIAL CYSTITIS

So here I sit, telling my story at thirty-nine years of age, knowing that someone out there is struggling with the same condition and in the same place I was several years ago. Struggling with how to live with and manage interstitial cystitis is a difficult place to be. I hope my story gives a sense of a future with this condition unmarked by long-term negativity. I also hope that those who do not have chronic conditions can gain a better understanding of the power that conditions like IC can have over a person's life. Maybe this story, and the story of so many others, will help us all be more sympathetic and encouraging.

While I hope my story helps others, telling it also helped me discover my personal growth gained from this experience. I know my body better now than I ever have. I am more understanding of others with varying conditions. I am humbled by the experience of having little control of my bodily functions and the work it took to gain that control back. In retrospect, I experienced a great deal of personal growth, which scholars call posttraumatic growth.

Posttraumatic growth (PTG) is a process that individuals go through where they show positive personal growth after the experience of a life-altering event (Zeligman, Varney, Grad, & Huffstead, 2018). Individuals who experience PTG can experience advantages such as positive physical and emotional health benefits, increase in coping abilities, and a greater sense of well-being. Zeligman and colleagues (2018) found that meaning making is one of the strongest predictors of posttraumatic growth. I have definitely experienced PTG. Knowing that I have gone through this entire process without naming it seems odd to me, especially as an academic. I knew what meaning making was (it was a portion of my dissertation), but I was not able to label it at the time it was happening. Yet this is all part of the human process we are all subject to. Now I can look back and see that the meaning I assigned to this experience was directly related to gaining control and independence of my healthcare. Withnall (2017) said it best in relation to her chronic illness, "I understand empowerment as the ability to identify, access and make use of the resources necessary to take control of my illness" (p. 475).

I started my journey with interstitial cystitis by allowing medical professionals to make decisions about what I needed. I did not educate myself on other possible avenues of care. I did not know that I could care for myself. Upon learning that I could have control over my body and my health, I turned a new leaf. My experiences with IC and varying medical practitioners taught me that I must be educated about my health to advocate for myself. My posttraumatic growth includes learning about myself, what I can handle, what I cannot cope with well, and how to advocate for myself, which has been invaluable. Dr. Adams showed me, in a few words and actions, that I had the power to let IC control me or take control of my life and allow interstitial cystitis to be one small part of a very awesome existence.

CONCLUSION

Until recently, I had not thought of interstitial cystitis as a chronic condition. I do not really know why; maybe it was a subconscious way of coping. When I finally accepted IC as being chronic, I was able to convince myself that I had to live with IC rather than just limiting myself to coping with it. This means not holding back on my relationship to the condition in the same way that I had been. Interstitial cystitis will always be part of my life but it controlled me for too long. I decided not to let it control me any longer. I will always think about my condition, how it will affect the activities I participate in, and those I choose not to. However, it cannot rule my life or ruin my life. Now I take more chances and care for myself in ways I never have before. I have been running regularly, which is a first since high school sports twenty years ago. I have lost the weight I gained from the time when I felt as if my body was not worth caring for. I am stronger in the hopes that the better condition my body is in, the better my mind will be, and the better I will be able to *live* with interstitial cystitis.

REFERENCES

Babrow, A. S., Kline, K. N., & Rawlins, W. K. (2005). Narrating problems and problematizing narratives: Linking problematic integration and narrative theory in telling stories about our health. In L. M. Harter, P. M. Japp, & C. S. Beck (Eds.), *Narratives, health and healing: Communication theory, research, and practice* (pp. 31–52). Mahwah, NJ: Lawrence Erlbaum Associates.

Bochner, A. P., & Ellis, C. S. (2006). Communication as autoethnography. In G. J. Shepherd, J. St. John, & T. Striphas (Eds.), *Communication as...Perspectives on theory* (pp. 110–22). Thousand Oaks, CA: Sage.

Ellis, C. S. (2004). *The ethnographic I: A methodological novel about autoethnography*. Walnut Creek, CA: AltaMira Press.

Ellis, C., Adams, T. E., & Bochner, A. P. (2011). Autoethnography: An overview. *Historical Social Research, 36* (4), 273–90.

Ettorre, E. (2016). *Autoethnography as feminist method: Sesitising the feminist 'I,'* London, England: Routledge.

Harp, L. M., Japp, P. M., & Beck, C. S. (2005). Problematics of narrative theorizing about health and healing. In L. M. Harter, P. M. Japp, & C. S. Beck (Eds.), *Narratives, health and healing: Communication theory, research, and practice* (pp. 31–52). Mahwah, NJ: Lawrence Erlbaum Associates.

Harter, L. M., & Bochner, A. P. (2009). Healing through stories: A special issue on narrative medicine. *Journal of Applied Communication Research, 37*(2), 113–17. DOI: 10.1082/00909880902792271.

Holman, H., & Lorig, K. (2000). Patients as partners in managing chronic disease: Partnership is a prerequisite for effective and efficient health care. *British Medical Journal, 320* (7234), 526–27.

Jago, B. J. (2002). Chronicling an academic depression. *Journal of Contemporary Ethnography, 31* (6), 729–57. DOI: 10.1177/089124102237823.

Kralik, D. (2002). The quest for ordinariness: Transition experienced by midlife women living with chronic illness. *Journal of Advanced Nursing, 39* (2), 146–54. DOI: 10.1046/j.1365-2648.2000.02254.x.

Mayo Clinic (2018a). *Endometriosis*. Retrieved from https://www.mayoclinic.org/diseases-conditions/endometriosis/symptoms-causes/syc-20354656.

Mayo Clinic (2018b). *Pelvic organ prolapse*. Retrieved from https://www.mayoclinic.org/diseases-conditions/pelvic-organ-prolapse/symptoms-causes/syc-20360557.

McGonagle, A. K., & Adams-Farrell, J. L. (2013). Chronic illness in the workplace: Stigma, identity threat and strain. *Stress Health, 30* (4), 310–21. DOI: 10.1002/smi.2518.

Richards, R. (2008). Writing the othered self: Autoethnography and the problem of objectification in writing about illness and disability. *Qualitative Research Reports, 18* (12), 1717–728. DOI: 10.1177/1049732308325866.

Ronai, C. R. (1992). Multiple reflections of child sex abuse. *Journal of Contemporary Ethnography, 23*, 395–425. DOI: 10.1177/089124195023004001.

Spieldenner, A. R. (2014). Statement of ownership: An autoethnography of living with HIV. *The Journal of Men's Studies, 22* (1), 12–27. DOI: 10.3149/jms.2201.12.

Webster, D. C. (1996). Sex, lies, and stereotypes: Women and interstitial cystitis. *The Journal of Sex Research, 33* (3), 197–203.

Withnall, A. (2017). Learning to live with chronic illness in later life: Empowering myself. *Australian Journal of Adult Learning, 57* (3), 474–89.

Zeligman, M., Varney, M., Grad, R. I., & Huffstead, M. (2018). Posttraumatic growth in individuals with chronic illness: The role of social support and meaning making. *Journal of Counseling & Development, 96* (1), 53–63. DOI: 10.1002/jcad.12177.

Chapter Eight

Narrating Menopause with English as a Second Language

Wei Sun

In November 2015, on a flight to Las Vegas for a national academic conference, I experienced a sudden, severe chest pain. *Should I check into a hospital as soon as we land? Should I call my family on the East Coast? Should I let my friends and colleagues who were attending the same conference know?* These thoughts immediately raced through my head and lingered for days afterward. However, by the end of the conference, I had not taken any of those actions. I thought the chest pain to be a false alarm; that no useful information would be gleaned from a medical examination.

When I came back home from the trip and finally made an appointment with my family doctor, she ran an electrocardiogram (ECG) test and immediately sent me to the ER. The ECG diagram chart showed that I had had two previous heart attacks. I was utterly shocked. Sitting in the ER that day, wires attached all over me and surrounded by beeping medical equipment, frenzied thoughts swirled through my mind. *Do I have heart disease? Is it caused by stress? Was it hereditary? What's next?*

Eventually, the doctors found no symptoms of heart disease, nor were they able to explain why the chest pain occurred. After hours of observation in the ER, the doctors released me with the advice to take Tylenol if the chest pain was intolerable. I felt some relief in the simple conclusion and prescribed treatment. But it was still bothersome that no root cause was found.

In years past, I had visited doctors in various specialties, and underwent outpatient treatments for perimenopause disorder. As I researched menopause, I discovered that the health complaints I had in recent years were all symptoms traceable to perimenopause or menopause. A seasonal change: a life change, a discomfort, and an unprepared and prolonged transition. According to the Mayo Clinic (2017), menopause marks the end of a woman's menstrual cycles and usually happens in her forties or fifties. The symptoms include hot flushes, sleep problems, emotional changes, irregular periods, and heart problems, to name a few. But without undergoing menopause themselves, few understand the lived reality of frustration, uncertainty, and the long-suffering present in this life phase.

Most women in my generation report discomfort related to physical change when they reach their forties and fifties. Those who are lucky experience little discomfort. The unlucky experience prolonged discomfort and suffering. It is a common health concern for people at menopause age (Mayo Clinic, 2017). Certain diseases are related to women during the menopausal phase, such as heart attack, stroke, and cancers (Dalai & Agarwal, 2015). Overcoming menopause seems to become a benchmark for a woman's longevity (White et al., 2015). While seeking treatments for my menopause-related "disorder," I realized there are often gaps between what a woman expects, what she actually experiences, and the reactions of her doctor, family members, and friends.

This chapter uses autoethnography and ethnographic interviews as research methods to investigate how women who speak English as a second language narrate their stories to others. The research will offer a deeper understanding of cultural competency in lifespan health communication contexts.

LITERATURE REVIEW

The following sections review literature on three topics: menopause, culture and quality of life; women's wellness, hormone treatment, and exercise during the menopausal phase; and narratives and empowerment discourse.

Menopause, Culture, and Quality of Life

Menopause creates many physical and emotional challenges to women in midlife (Amonkar & Mody, 2002; Avis et al., 2004; Delanoë et al., 2012; Henderson et al., 2008; Kripke et al., 2004; Llaneza et al., 2012; Shukla, Ganjiwale, & Patel, 2018). Melby, Lock, and Kaufert (2005) have studied how women from different countries and ethnicities report menopause symptoms. Menopause "is understood as a process, part of the phenomenon of aging, and is associated with both social and biological changes" (p. 500). Cross-cultural research on menopause indicates that very few women experience menopause with long-term discomfort. Foci of the studies of women in different countries have been on the average age when the transition occurs, family history, and physical and mental symptoms related to the life changes (Llaneza et al., 2012). Taking a lifespan approach, scholars believe that when considering menopause, it is important to combine genetics, environment, culture, social economic status, and lifestyle together (Leidy, 1994; Llanza et al., 2012; Melby & Lamp, 2011). Certain menopause symptoms might be influenced by discordance of lifestyle changes and genetic heritage, such as migration and diet change (Melby & Lamp, 2011).

Research studies on relationships between women's quality of life and menopause show that depression is commonly experienced (Li & Holm, 2003; Simon et al., 2013; Harvard Medical School, 2006). Researchers suggest that increased physical activity and individualized coping strategies are important to help women overcome negative attitudes toward aging and menopause (Derry, 2004; Hwang et al., 2016). Firquet, Kirschner, and Bitzer (2017) study the iron deficiency anemia among women in menopause ages and point out that untreated anemia leads to fatigue, which has a negative impact on women's quality of life.

Mazahery, Stonehouse, and von Hurst (2015) prescribe high dosages of vitamin D to immigrant women at menopause age to treat vitamin D deficiency and bolster energy. Shufelt (2017), who studies heart disease in midlife women, warns that middle-aged women usually have persistent atypical and mild symptoms compared to men who have heart disease, and thus have lower rates of heart disease diagnosis and higher rates of death.

Allsworth and associates (2004) investigate relations between the timing and violence women experienced in childhood and adulthood to menopause timings. They find that life course accelerates to menopause transitions. Life situations including traumas have been found to accelerate a woman's transition to menopause (Allsworth et al., 2004). Several studies have focused on the impact of life events on women's menopausal depression. Women who experience disease and who lose family members are more likely to develop depression and low self-esteem (Schmidt et al., 2004).

Woods and Mitchell (2005) further study the symptoms during perimenopause and the significance of the prevalence and severity in women's lives. They propose that women may have experienced more severe symptoms when dealing with daily living demands and maintenance of different roles in family and the workplace. Other researchers have also studied menopausal distress, anxiety, and anxiety sensitivity from the perspectives of biopsychosocial characteristics and personality traits (Muslic and Jokic-Begic, 2016; Morgan et al., 2012), and urge medical professionals to intervene with health education and for women to practice healthful behaviors (Tsao et al., 2007; Eun, 2006; Morgan et al., 2012; Angın, Erden, & Can, 2015).

WOMEN'S WELLNESS, HORMONE TREATMENT, AND PHYSICAL EXERCISE DURING THE MENOPAUSAL PHASE

Women across the world experience menopause as a challenge to women's wellness, and the idea of hormone therapy has become an option (Anderson et al., 2004; Gupta, Sturdee, & Hunter, 2006; Jones et al., 2012; Kripke et al., 2004). Klaiber, Vogel, and Rako (2005) review the women's health initiative in hormone therapy and argue that hormone therapy might be beneficial in women with cardiovascular symptoms during menopause. However, younger women in perimenopause stages receive greater benefit compared to women at later stages of menopause (Hansson, Hedner, & Himmelmann, 2000). In the United Kingdom, scientists conducted a One Million Women study that found correlations between hormone usage and incidences of breast cancer. While the overall results show the positive effect of using the hormone, observational studies indicate that certain risks like breast, ovarian, endometrial, and colorectal cancers correlates to usage (Barret, 2001). Archibald and colleagues (2006) studied breast cancer survivors and found that chemical induced menopause and its side effects create extra stressors for affected women. The side effects include lack of sexual desire and lower self-esteem due to anxiety and depression as a result of treatment.

Ascott-Evans and co-researchers (2003) observe a high rate of bone strength loss in the first year after discontinuation of hormone replacement treatment among postmenopausal women. According to their study, 30 to 50 percent of women will suffer a severe fracture within their lives. Seventy percent of hip fracture patients are women. It has been proven that hormone replacement therapy could reduce all osteoporosis-related fractures by 30 percent (Ascott-Evans et al., 2003). Balabanovic, Ayers, and Hunter (2013) recognize the growing need for medically noninvasive treatments for menopausal women experiencing hot flushes and night sweats. In a qualitative study investigating the quality of life of women experiencing menopause related symptoms, Ayers, and Hunter (2013) identified four themes that include understanding the symptom change, learning to cope and control, breaking the taboo of menopause, and using social support and personal learning. If women receive sufficient information about the physical and emotional change during menopause phase, it becomes easier for them to accept the change (Ayers & Hunter, 2013).

Karacan (2010) examines the long-term effects of aerobic exercise on physical fitness and postmenopausal symptoms and believes that women who exercise regularly and intensively are more likely to stay fit and have fewer menopausal symptoms. Sharma and Mahajan (2015) compare menopausal women in Indian rural and urban areas and assert women from both rural and urban settings all report high rates of menopausal symptoms. However, while women from rural areas suffer higher severity of symptoms, their measurement of quality of life scored lower than women from urban areas.

Eun and her colleagues (2010) conducted a national study on menopausal symptoms among four major ethnic groups (White, Black, Hispanic, and Asian) in the United States. The qualitative research categorizes common characteristics across the ethnic groups, such as levels of optimism, availability of support, and access to information to understand menopause is just a life process. Even though the research is unable to distinguish the differences among groups, it does emphasize the empowerment of women with midlife challenges. Stefanopoulou and her colleagues (2014) conducted an international study of climate, altitude, and temperature effects on women's menopause. They found that women who have poorer general health tend to have more negative beliefs regarding menopause and that women who exercise less tend to have more severe menopausal symptoms. The study concludes that factors such as health condition, mood, health beliefs, and lifestyles can explain some of the menopausal symptoms. Matthews and her colleagues (2002) assessed the body mass index in a multiethnic sample of mid-life women between ages forty and fifty-five at seven sites, including 7,181 Caucasians, 3,949 African Americans, 1,660 Hispanics, and 1,365 Eastern Asians. The study found that inactive women with a higher BMI tend to report surgical menopause, an unnatural aging process caused by a surgery to remove the ovaries. Physical activity is beneficial for health promotion and disease prevention in the general population, however, less than half of the population exercises regularly. Very few women from ages forty to sixty maintain even minimal physical activities (Sternfeld & Dugan, 2011). Researchers recommend that women increase physical activity to prevent common weight gain during menopause (Beard et al., 2016; Poyatos & Abellán, 2011).

Narratives and Empowerment Discourse

Vinson (2016) studies patient empowerment discourse, and suggests that "active patienthood is normatively good, and that patients should inform themselves, claim their expertise, and participate in their care" (p. 1364). She advocates for a constrained collaboration to encourage interactions between patients and physicians. Wentzer and Bygholm (2013) study narratives of online community patient support groups and recognize the importance of patient empowerment at the individual level and compliance of doctor's recommendation at the collective level. In a Quit Smoking research study, Kim and his associates (2012) explored the psychological impact of narrative on behavioral intention. Study results found that when reading information about quitting smoking, the more a reader engages with the narratives, the greater the impact on the intention to quit smoking.

In a healthcare context, physician-patient relationships have been regarded as a critical factor in medical information interview, diagnosis, and decision making on treatment plans (Ha & Longnecker, 2010). Even though communication effectiveness between a physician and a patient is valued, misunderstanding can always occur. The doctor-patient relationship has been neglected in professional training among doctors (Chandra, Mohammadnezhad, & Ward, 2018; Comaroff, 1976; Goold & Lipkin, 1999; Strong, 2012), especially for people who speak English as a second language who must overcome language barriers and cultural barriers when contacting medical providers (Strong, 2012; Sun, 2017). Social support and information sharing among their own linguistic communities is usually the way people find health information and that information is sometimes partial or even untrue (Moreno, Otero-Sabogal, & Newman, 2007). Tracy and associates (2004) examined patient decision making regarding disclosure of personal health information among people who speak English as a second language and found that most participants had expressed mistrust regarding how their information might be used.

Research has confirmed that menopause creates health and emotional challenges for women across all ethnicities. However, few have addressed the concerns of women who speak English as a second language. In dealing with menopausal symptoms, how do they narrate their experiences to doctors, families, and friends? How do they get help? The central questions are: What are the physical and emotional challenges English as a second language (ESL) women in menopause experience? How do ESL women narrate and relate their symptoms/experiences to doctors and others? And what social and emotional support exists for ESL menopausal women's needs?

THEORETICAL FRAMEWORK AND METHODS

A culture-centered approach to health communication is used as a theoretical framework. In his research on marginalized communication practices in healthcare settings, Dutta (2007) proposes that culture should be the center of the communication process, and that cultural participants should co-construct the meanings in health contexts. Identity constructions, sense-making, and life experiences should be the highlights in health communication. The culture-centered approach gives voice to cultural members in co-construction of health risks faced by the community. Listening to their voices will help health institutions fully understand the problems members of underrepresented groups face so that in the future, policy-making and intervention can be implemented in a culture centered and appropriate dimension. In this chapter, I use an autoethnography method and ethnographic interviews to investigate women's menopausal experiences.

Autoethnography has been used in qualitative research to describe and understand cultural experiences (Ellis & Bochner, 2006; 2000). Bochner (2012) argues that autoethnography builds a rapport relationship between the storyteller and the story listener and encourages conversations through "the heartbreaking feelings of stigma and marginalization . . . the therapeutic desire to face up to the challenges of life and to emerge with greater self-knowledge, the opposition to the repression of the body, the difficulty of finding the words to make bodily dysfunction meaningful" (p. 159). Analytic autoethnography not only provides personal reflections, but also analyzes and generalizes data so as to stimulate theoretical development, refinement, extension, and encourage further conversation. Autoethnographers can create and structure narratives in different formats. One is co-constructed narratives: this format "illustrate[s] the meanings of relational experiences, particularly how people collaboratively cope with the ambiguities, uncertainties, and contradictions about some aspect of their relations, often told about or around an epiphany" (Ellis & Bochner, 2006, p. 279). Epiphany is defined by Kien (2013) as "an identifiable moment of lived experience that one can identify as a turning point in one's understanding of oneself and one's relationship to the world . . . the epiphany compels the researcher to return to and explore that life-altering moment." (p. 578). Kien (2013) encourages ethnographers to always return to the moments, reexamine the epiphanies, and interpret the deeper meanings behind them.

Ethnography focuses on complex "descriptions of a culture-sharing group . . . the culture sharing group must have been intact and interacting to develop social behaviors of an identifiable group that can be studied" (Creswell & Poth, 2018, p. 91). An ethnographic research study will explore patterns through language and activities of the group. Through observations, interviews, and listening, the researcher "asks the right questions in the right way" (Westby, Burda, & Mehta, 2003, p. 4).

In this chapter, relational ethics is used to give readers an understanding of the cultural aspects involved in the menopausal experience of women for whom English is their second language (ESL). I invite readers to be co-participants as the stories are told. Through the reader's own interpretations of the stories of ESL women, cultural understanding could potentially be achieved to allow them to make sense of why menopausal symptoms are challenging for ESL women (Ellis & Bochner, 2006; Sun, 2017). For this study, I recruited and interviewed ten Asian American women through a snowball sampling from a social network. We all speak English as a second language, and our native language is Mandarin. The ages of those in the group range from fifty to sixty-one. Participants all came to the United States in their thirties. As a researcher and participant who experienced menopausal symptoms, it made my approach to participants easier. A rapport relationship was established to ensure openness to the topic. Throughout the semi-structured interviews conducted both in Chinese and English, participants chose to speak either or both languages. I translated the Chinese into English, and offered member checking with the participants to warrant the accuracy of data (Harper & Cole, 2012; Rager, 2005). (See table 8.1 for participants' demographics.)

Table 8.1. Participants' Demographics

	Age	Marital Status	Education	Menopause Age	Past Health History	Job Status
YM	51	divorced	B.S.	48		IT engineer
AC	55	divorced	M.S.	50	breast cancer	researcher
AB	50s	married	B.A.	51		manager
GN	55	divorced	Ph.D.	48	hypertension	faculty
NN	55	married	Vocational	47	colorectal cancer	school cashier
UI	61	divorced	Ph.D.	51	colorectal cancer	early retirement
CW	50s	married	B.A.	50	thyroid cancer	teacher assistant
SN	52	separate	Ph.D.	48	hyperthyroidism	college instructor
XS	52	separate	M.S.	47		lab technician
AU	55	divorced	MA	48	heart disease	stay home writer

NARRATIVE THEMES FOR ESL WOMEN IN MENOPAUSE

Using a systematic approach of grounded theory introduced by Glasser and Stauss (1999), I examined the transcripts from the interviews and the notes from my own critical moments. The following thematic issues emerged from data and the discussions:

Embarrassing Moments Hindered Social Interactions and Relationships

Menopausal incidents oftentimes catch women in unexpected places and times. Due to fear, women with menopausal symptoms may feel the necessity to constrain their physical and social activities. There are women, including myself, who are afraid to "lose face" in public, and chose to hide from others.

> I was irritated by invitations for social functions. "What if something happens just like last time?" Once at the church after the Sunday service, sitting in the first row of chairs, I felt the familiar blood draining, and the pants and the chair I was sitting on soaked immediately. That was supposed to be the last day of

the menstrual cycle. I was not prepared for the heavy bleeding. Actually even when prepared, there is no way to prevent the disaster. At the end of the service, I whispered to my neighbor, "I cannot move." Knowing I have had the problem for years, she went to the restroom, and got me a roll of toilet paper . . . nobody can imagine how embarrassed I was. For weeks after that incident, I didn't even want to see anyone from the church. —WS

AB, who has suffered from menopausal symptoms since she was fifty-one, describes her experience as follows:

> Since I started to have menopause, I have constantly spotty [sic] and bleeding all year around. It not only has caused anemia in me, I feel weak and fragile all the time. I have passed out at work, which scared my colleagues to death. . . . This has become a serious issue with my spouse, and of course, our intimate relationship has been affected. —AB

Looking at the participants' demographics, I acknowledge that four are cancer survivors, five were divorced, two are separating, and one is single. Very few made connections that menopausal symptoms might correlate with cancer or other illness, or that it could impact their relationships. Participant OI admitted that she could not tell if the symptoms and discomfort she experienced at the time was related to menopause or a side effect of the chemotherapy. In their narratives, the other three cancer survivors never connected the dots that they were diagnosed with cancer at the same time of the menopausal phase. However, according to Dalai and Agarwal (2015), cancer is related to menopausal women, and menopause could impact women's life quality significantly (Simon et al., 2013). Among the single and separated women, no one thought that menopause might impact intimate relationships. Only one woman was actively seeking a dating partner at the time of interview. She complained:

> I never expect [sic] that my period to stop all of a sudden. Since I was forty-nine, I have experienced an irregular period, sweating, and mood swings. I went to the doctor and she prescribed me progesterone to regulate the period. The first time I took it, I had a [sic] heavy bleeding for seven days. Then the period never came back. I still feel young and since I'm at the beginning of my new relationship, this hits me so hard. I feel that being a woman, my feminine self is taken away with the period. —YM

Doctor Visits, Treatment, and Procedures

It is widely accepted that communicating with doctors could be a problem for patients who speak English as a second language (Moreno, Otero-Sabogal, & Newman, 2007; Strong, 2012; Sun, 2017). In ethnographic interviews, very few admit that seeing an English-speaking doctor is a problem. The reason might be that my participants are highly educated. Except for one person who has a vocational degree, two have bachelor's degrees, and the others have graduate degrees. Having been in this country (United States) for a long time, many know what to expect from an English-speaking-only doctor. In my own experience, even though I do not mind going to English-speaking-only doctors, if possible, I still prefer a Mandarin-speaking doctor. Then I can use my native language to say the hard pronouncing jargon words such as hemorrhage, hematoma, hysterectomy, and endometritis.

Even though most of the participants say they have no difficulty in communicating with their English-speaking-only doctors, few of them reported getting valuable treatments or advice regarding how to cope with menopausal symptoms. Among participants, three of them work in medical fields and believe specialists in their own network or information found by themselves. Their narratives are in accordance with previous researches that ESL patients do not trust medical professionals. They often rely on themselves and in-group sharing for generating medical knowledge (Balabanovic, Ayers, & Hunter, 2013; Moreno, Otero-Sabogal, & Newman, 2007; Sun, 2017).

> I had two surgeries during my menopause. One is related to menopause, another is a different health issue. I took my doctors' advice, but it did not relieve the symptoms. Later, I think American doctors' levels are just so-so, I did some research to try to be my own doctor. —GN

> I saw several gynecologists when I had hemorrhage and hematoma. I have no problem telling them in English. They seem to understand my problems and have sympathy for me. But they can't do anything to help me. So far, I still suffer the symptoms. —AB

> My doctor told me menopause is a process. For some, it is prolonged, for others it might be short. She recommended me [sic] to take hormone treatment, let me do ultrasounds, and check the blood for the hormone. She did everything she could do. She even consulted her colleagues, but they can't explain why my period stops, but my hormone level is normal. —YM

> In the middle of 2010s [sic], I frequently visited doctors for my menopause symptoms. My family doctor recommended me [sic] to see a male Chinese gynecologist; he performed the C&D [sic] in his Clinic. I chose to see an English-speaking doctor whose online reviews were good. It turns out she also sees people with various addictions. I felt weird to see many men visiting a gynecologist's office. Even though when I spoke to her, she seems to have the right expertise. While waiting for a medical procedure with this doctor, I had a hemorrhage twice in a row and passed out due to anemia. I was sent to the ER and was referred to a first available gynecologist. He performed a surgery on me, and it was successful. But unfortunately, he relocated to a different health system my insurance did not cover. From then I haven't had a gynecologist. Among all the gynecologists I had seen, this is the most qualified doctor.

English is his second language also. But he has cultural understanding, sympathizes to women [sic] in the menopausal phase, listens patiently to my health history, and has excellent expertise, knowledge, and skills. —WS

I feel communicating to a doctor is difficult because, first, I needed to describe some symptoms related to sex life and private life and that makes me uncomfortable. Second, I am not sure how much other people revealed their symptoms in their doctor visits—I didn't want to go to great details, but didn't want to hide needed information from my doctor unnecessarily. And third, there were some terminologies that the doctor did not try to explain plainly and I was too shy to ask for elaboration. —SN

Mood Swaying, Stress, and Other Health Complaints

Women in the menopausal phase often feel tired, stressed, depressed, and bothered by other health issues (Llaneza et al., 2012; Shukla, Ganjiwale, & Patel, 2018). Hot flushes, sweating, mood swaying, and disturbed sleeping are commonly perceived by participants in this study. While women in menopause deal with declining health, they are often still working full time in their own professions, providing for the family, and maintaining relationships. Work-related stress combines with health issues and family obligation to cast extreme burdens on participants. According to studies, there is a significant connection between work related stress and health outcomes (The American Institution of Stress, 2017; Sun, 2019). I was teaching at three colleges one semester right after a surgery. Walking from the parking lot to the classroom would make me out of breath. I dared not take a break as I was preparing for a promising job. After I started a tenure-track position at a research university, I quit all other teaching jobs. To deal with new challenges and demands, I work extra hard, go to every grant workshop, sit on committees, and write proposal after proposal . . . I cannot tell the truth to my family and friends in China about why at middle age, I have started as an assistant professor while my peers in China are retiring from the workforce. It was right after my new job started when I was diagnosed with sleep apnea. Many mornings I drove to school feeling dizzy and I was constantly yawning in meetings due to the poor quality of sleep. I cannot tell my deans why I kept yawning. It does not seem acceptable by workplace standards to ask for leave for menopausal related illnesses.

CW's menopause seems okay. She told me a story of her friend, who works as a realtor who experienced swaying moods.

> I have a friend who is a realtor who I have known for years. She told me she needs to see a psychiatrist. While she was driving, her eyelids drooped. She had to use one hand to drive and the other hand to keep her eyes open. But she often fell asleep while driving. One day she woke up finding herself parked in a stranger's driveway! Sometimes she would drive like a manic, screaming

and shouting like a crazy woman. She said that then she would feel better. That was when I was in my late thirties. She said she was having menopause. She kept asking me if she was insane. I felt she had too much pressure from life, and her family members did not comfort her. I had a fear of menopause. —CW

GN, a college professor, feels she is easily provoked all the time, and she notices her emotional and physical change during menopause but feels hopeless in "controlling" it. As a single mom, she has a child in college who needs her financial support; as research faculty, she is stressed out often at the workplace. In her words:

I just hope I am healthy and get over with this stage. I have lots of things to do. My aging parents in China also need my support. Even though I feel I am on the edge of breaking down, I have no one to depend on and I have to be strong. —GN

Another participant, SN, a college instructor, is virtually separated from her husband. Her husband stays in China while she is teaching, and their only child is in college. She had passed out several times during her perimenopause phase due to heavy menstrual bleeding. Fortunately, both times she was attended to. Once it happened in a relative's house, another time during a quarrel with her husband. When she was diagnosed with hyperthyroid, she said she often felt her moods are like a roller-coaster. She could not hold her anger and she usually ended up saying something destructive that later she would regret. She was afraid to take medicine for the rest of her life. For the first month, she took the prescription drug for controlling hyperthyroid, it then developed into hyperthyroidism. She wonders from time to time if she should continue to take the pills or reduce the amount of the pills she takes.

Social and Emotional Support

Oftentimes, women from underrepresented groups have health issues and face the challenges with little to no social and emotional support due to cultural taboos, sometimes due to personalities, oftentimes due to the nature of the illness (Madlock Gatison, 2016; Sun, 2017). Diseases related to women are often not publicly discussed in front of men, or younger women. In my own case, I seek out female friends who are at a similar age and who have similar experiences. We exchange medical information such as which gynecologist is trustworthy, what medicine we are taking, and what procedures we have had.

Often feeling depressed, YM feels better after talking to others. Especially after she knows other people also experience menopausal symptoms. That helps her reduce anxiety. AU also feels better when she speaks to friends, receiving comfort from others. NN would encourage others to relax and not overthink too much. Be happy, then it will be over soon. SN states:

> I have talked to some close friends about the symptoms. The talks did help in that I learned I was not alone feeling that way, and I should not be blamed or blame myself. Because I was undergoing some physical change my family members and colleagues had no way to understand themselves. When I talked to friends who were experiencing the same stage, their sharing was especially supportive and beneficial to me. Other friends would give me advice, comfort me, and prayed with me when necessary. —SN

There are also those who do not talk to anyone about the problems, such as AC, UI, AB, GN, and CW. They do not think talking to others will help at all. AB said she had talked to others before but felt it was useless. She says she would rather look for information on her own. There is an absence of spousal or partner support from all participants, except CW. CW is the only one who says her relationships with others became better. Even though she is reluctant to refer to with whom she has had a better relationship. In the Chinese language, both "him" and "her" are pronounced as "ta," which is gender undistinguishable unless written down.

DISCUSSION

While menopausal symptoms create physiological discomfort and beat down the spirits, the most worrisome issues for these Chinese American women at menopausal phase are:

First, the lack of standard procedures for women to look for medical information and help. This is a very well educated and well-informed group. If for them the proper care and treatment are difficult to find, it must be more difficult for other people who do not have similar resources. Women must actively seek out needed information, credible doctors, and effective treatments (Melby, Lock, & Kaufert, 2005). In most cases, there is no successful formula besides passive waiting: waiting for the symptoms to be over, waiting for the next doctor to be a specialist, waiting for the timing to be over as soon as possible. Among Asian American women, health disparities are present not only for low social-economic class but also for the middle class. This echoes recent research on Asian American health disparities. For African American and Hispanics, health disparities exist for those on the lower end of the social-economic spectrum. But for Asian Americans, no matter if low or high in social-economic status, health outcomes do not always match their social-economic status (Mui et al., 2017; Yu, Huang, & Singh, 2010).

Second, there is an absence of spousal support in these stories. For participating women, their social and emotional support are mainly from other women who also are experiencing similar menopausal symptoms. In previous research on cancer, I have specified that "the relationships and support systems which are considered key aspects in cancer patients' survivorship barely exist for Chinese American cancer patients" (Sun, 2017, p. 135). It is also true for menopausal Chinese American women. The Chinese culture is "a collective, highly contextual, and gender-specific culture" (Sun, 2017, p. 135). Men do not usually directly show affection. Therefore, professional Chinese American women become more independent and do not rely on men. This creates the impression that men are absent. None of the married participants said that their spouse provides emotional support.

Third, stress may have intensified participating women's menopausal discomfort. The stress experienced at work and at home seems to add to the burden of the participating women. The American Institution of Stress reports in 2017, 80 percent of employees reported work-related stress and 29 percent report experiencing burnout from work. Job-related stress has surpassed the stress caused by financial and personal issues. Job-related stress has a high correlation with health complaints, low morale, disruption, and high turnover rates (Sun, 2019). Menopause is a life-changing event, which could trigger more stress for women.

CONCLUSION

This study helps to support the idea that health professionals should develop culturally appropriate and cultural centered competencies in providing health care to patients who speak English as a second language. Particularly important are competencies in understanding how women, whose first language and culture of origin is not English speaking, narrate their experiences based on where they are from and what language is their primary one. As part of these narrative competencies, doctors might be more mindful of listening well, and even spending more time when seeing an ESL patient. It can be difficult for women who speak English as a second language to seek professional help, and more skillful narrative engagement might help. On the other side of the care (and communication) relationship, ESL patients might more actively seek information from each other (patient narrative sharing), and self-study the medical literacy (informed narration). Similarly, improving their ability to narrate their experiences by using more direct communication styles to specify how they feel and what they are experiencing might improve caregiver-patient communication. Such narrative skills on both sides help, but there is a long way to go, and more narrative research is needed to more fully understand and enable adaptation to the communication needs of various groups of patients who live in the United States and who speak English as a second language.

REFERENCES

Allsworth, J. E., Zierter, S., Lapane, K., & Krieger, N. (2004). Longitudinal study of the of the inception of perimenopaise in relation to lifetime history of sexual or physical violence. *Journal of epidemiology and community health, 58,* 11: 938–943.

Amonkar, M. M., & Mody, R. (2002). Developing profiles of postmenopausal women being prescribed estrogen therapy to prevent osteoporosis. *Journal of Community Health, 27*(5), 335–51.

Anderson, D., Yoshizawa, T., Gollschewski, S., Atogami, F., & Courtney, M. (2004). Menopause in Australia and Japan: effects of country of residence on menopausal status and menopausal symptoms. *Climacteric, 7*(2), 165–74.

Angın, E., Erden, Z., & Can, F. (2015). The effects of clinical pilates exercises on bone mineral density, physical performance and quality of life of women with postmenopausal osteoporosis. *Journal of Back & Musculoskeletal Rehabilitation, 28*(4), 849–58.

Archibald, S., Lemieux, S., Byers, E. S., Tamlyn, K., & Worth, J. (2006). Chemically-Induced Menopause and the Sexual Functioning of Breast Cancer Survivors. *Women & Therapy, 29*(1/2), 83–106.

Ascott-Evans, B. H., Guañabens, N., Kivinen, S., Stuckey, B. G. A., Magaril, C. H., Vandormael, K . . . Melton, M. E. (2003). Alendronate Prevents Loss of Bone Density Associated With Discontinuation of Hormone Replacement Therapy: A Randomized Controlled Trial. *Archives of Internal Medicine, 163*(7), 789–95.

Avis, N. E., Assmann, S. F., Kravitz, H.M. Ganz, P. A., & Ory, M. (2004). Quality of life in diverse groups of midlife women: assessing the influence of menopause, health status and psychosocial and demographic factors. *Quality of Life Research, 13*(5), 933–46.

Ayers, B., & Hunter, M.S.(2013). Health-related quality of life of women with menopausal hot flushes and night sweats. *Climacteric,16*(2), 235–39.

Balabanovic, J., Ayers, B. & Hunter, M. S. (2013). Cognitive behaviour therapy for menopausal hot flushes and night sweats: A qualitative analysis of women's experiences of group and self-help CBT. *Behavioural & Cognitive Psychotherapy, 41*(4), 441–57.

Barret, J. R. (2001). A Million Women Get Hormonal. *Environmental Health Perspectives, 109*(8), p. A366.

Beard, J. R., Officer, A., de Carvalho, I. A., Sadana, R., Pot, A. M., Michel, J. P. . . . Chatterji, S. (2016). The World report on ageing and health: A policy framework for healthy ageing. *The Lancet, 387,* 10033, 2145–154.

Bochner, A. P. (2012). On first-person narrative scholarship: Autoethnography as acts of meaning. *Narrative Inquiry, 22*(1), 155–64.

Chandra, S., Mohammadnezhad, M., & and Ward, P. (2018). Trust and communication in a doctor patient relationship: A literature Review. *Journal of Healthcare Communications, 3*(3), 106.

Comaroff, J. (1976). Communicating information about non-fatal illness: The strategies of a group of general practictioners. *Sociological Review, 24*(2), 269–90.

Cresswell, J. W., & Poth, C. N. (2018, 5th edition). *Qualitative inquiry and research design: Choosing among five approaches.* Thousand Oaks, CA: Sage.

Dalai, P. K., & Agarwal,M. (2015) Postmenopausal syndrome. *Indian Journal of Psychiatry, 57*(2), S222–32.

Delanoë, D., Hajri, S., Bachelot, A., Mahfoudh, D. D., Hassoun, D., Marsicano, E., & Ringa, V. (2012). Class, gender and culture in the experience of menopause. A comparative survey in Tunisia and France. *Social Science & Medicine, 75*(2), 401–9.

Derry, P. S. (2004). Coping with Distress During Perimenopause. *Women & Therapy, 27*(3/4), 165–77.

Dutta, M.J. (2007). Communicating about culture and health: Theorizing culture-centered and cultural sensitivity approaches. *Communication Theory, 17*(3), 304–28.

Ellis, C., & Bochner, A. P. (2000). Autoethnography, personal narrative, reflexivity. In K. Denzin & Y. S. Lincoln (Eds.), *Handbook of qualitative research* (2nd ed., pp. 733–68). Thousand Oaks, CA: Sage.

Ellis, C. & Bochner, A.P. (2006). Analyzing analytic autoethnography: An autopsy. *Journal of Contemporary Ethnography, 35*(4), 429–49.

Eun, O. I. (2006). The Midlife Women's Symptom Index (MSI), *Health Care for Women International, 27*(3), 268–87.

Eun, O. I. , Bokim, L, Wonshik, C, Dormire, S., & Brown, A. (2010). A National Multiethnic Online Forum Study on Menopausal Symptom Experience. *Nursing Research Journal, 59*(1), 26–33.

Firquet, A., Kirschner, W., & Bitzer, J. (2017). Forty to fifty-five-year-old women and iron deficiency: clinical considerations and quality of life. *Gynecological Endocrinology, 33*(7), 503–9.

Glaser, B. G., & Strauss, A. L. (1999). Discovery of Grounded Theory. New York: Routledge.

Goold, S. D., & Lipkin, M. Jr. (1999). The doctor-patient relationship: Challenges, opportunities, and strategies. *Journal of General Internal Medicine, 14*(1), S26–S33.

Gupta, P., Sturdee, D. W., & Hunter, M. S. (2006). Mid-age health in women from the Indian subcontinent (MAHWIS): general health and the experience of menopause in women. *Climacteric, 9*(1), 13–22.

Ha, J. F., & Longnecker, N. (2010). Doctor-patient communication: a review. *The Ochsner journal, 10*(1), 38–43.

Hansson, L, Hedner, T., & Himmelmann, A. (2000). Postmenopausal Hormone Replacement Therapy and Hypertension. *Blood Pressure, 9*(5), 245.

Harper, M., & Cole, P. (2012). Member Checking: Can Benefits Be Gained Similar to Group Therapy? *The Qualitative Report, 17*(2), 510–17.

Harvard Medical School. (2006). Perimenopause, hormones, and midlife health. *Harvard Women's Health Watch, 14*(3), 1–3.

Henderson, K. D., Bernstein, L., Henderson, B., Kolonel, L., & Pike, M.C. (2008). Predictors of the timing of the natural menopause in the Multiple ethnic cohort study. *American Journal of Epidemiology, 167*(11), 1287–294.

Hwang, R.J, Wu, H. Y, Chen, H. J., & Yan, Y. J. (2016). Effect of exercise on the auditory discrimination task in perimenopausal women: a preliminary study. *Climacteric, 19*(3), 268–73.

Jones, E. K., Jurgenson, J. R., Katzenellenbogen, J. M., & Thompson, S. C. (2012). Menopause and the influence of culture: another gap for Indigenous Australian women? *BMC Women's Health, 12*(1), 43–52.

Karacan, S. (2010). Effects of long-term aerobic exercise on physical fitness and postmenopausal symptoms with menopausal rating scale. *Science & Sports, 25*(1), 39–46.

Kien, G. (2013). The nature of epiphany. *International Review of Qualitative Research, 6*(4), 578–84.

Kim, H. S., Bigman, C. A., Leader, A. E. Lerman, C., & Capella, J. N. (2012). Narrative Health Communication and Behavior Change: The Influence of Exemplars in the News on Intention to Quit Smoking. *Journal of Communication, 62*(3), 473–92.

Klaiber, E. L., Vogel, W., & Rako, S. (2005). A critique of the women's health initiative hormone therapy study. *Fertility & Sterility, 84*(6), 1589–601.

Kripke, D. F., Jean-Louis, G., Elliott, J. A., Klauber, M. R., Rex, K. M., Tuunainen, A., & Langer, R. D. (2004). Ethnicity, sleep, mood, and illumination in postmenopausal women. *BMC Psychiatry, 4*, 8–15.

Leidy, L.E. (1994). Biological aspects of menopause across the lifespan. *Annual Review of Anthropology, 23*, 231–252.

Li, S., & Holm, K. (2003). Physical activity alone and in combination with Hormone Replacement Therapy on vasomotor symptoms in postmenopausal women. *Western Journal of Nursing Research, 25*(3), 274–88.

Llaneza, P., García-Portilla, M., Llaneza-Suárez, D., Armott, B., & Pérez-López, F. R. (2012). Depressive disorders and the menopause transition. *Maturitas*, *71*(2), 120–30.

Madlock Gatison, A. D. (2016). *Health communication and breast cancer among Black women: Culture, identity, spirituality and strength.* Lanham, MD: Lexington Books.

Matthews, K. A., Abrams, B., Crawford, S., Miles, T., Neer, R., Powell, L. H., & Wesley, D. (2002). Body mass index in mid-life women: relative influence of menopause, hormone use, and ethnicity. *International Journal of Obesity*, *26*, 863–73.

Mayo Clinic (2017). Menopause. Retrieved from https://www.mayoclinic.org/diseases-conditions/menopause/symptoms-causes/syc-20353397.

Mazahery, H., Stonehouse, W. & von Hurst, P R. (2015). The effect of monthly 50 000 IU or 100 000 IU vitamin D supplements on vitamin D status in premenopausal Middle Eastern women living in Auckland European. *Journal of Clinical Nutrition*, *69*(3), 367–72.

Melby, M.K., & Lamp, M. (2011). Menopause, a biocultural perspective. *Annual Review of Anthropology*, *40*, 53–70.

Melby, M. K., Lock, M., & Kaufert, P. (2005). Culture and symptom reporting at menopause. *Human Reproduction Update*, *11*(5), 495–512.

Moreno, M. R., Otero-Sabogal, R., & Newman, J. (2007). Assessing Dual-role staff-interpreter linguistic competency in an integrated healthcare system. *Journal of General Internal Medicine*, *22*(2), 331–35.

Morgan, P., Merrell, J., Rentschler, D. & Chadderton, H. (2012). Uncertainty during perimenopause: perceptions of older first-time mothers. *Journal of Advanced Nursing*, *68*(10), 2299–308.

Mui, P., Bowie, J. V., Juon, H-S., & Thorpe, R. J. (2017). Ethnic group differences in health outcome among Asian American men in California. *American Journal of Men's Health*. *11*(5), 1406–414.

Muslić, L., & Jokić-Begić, N. (2016). The experience of perimenopausal distress: examining the role of anxiety and anxiety sensitivity. *Journal of Psychosomatic Obstetrics & Gynecology*, *37*(1), 26–33.

Poyatos, M.C. & Abellán, M. V. (2011). Training in a shallow pool: Its effect on upper extremity strength and total body weight in postmenopausal women. *International Sport Med Journal*, *12*(1), 17–29.

Rager, K. B. (2005). Self-care and the qualitative researcher: when collecting data can break your heart. Educational Researcher, 34(4), 23–27.

Schmidt, P. J., Haq, N., & Rubinow, D. R. (2004). A longitudinal evaluation of the relationship between reproductive status and mood in menopausal women. *American Journal of Psychiatry*, *12*: 22383–44.

Sharma, S., & Mahajan, N. (2015). Menopausal symptoms and its effect on quality of life in urban versus rural women: A cross-sectional study. *Journal of Mid-life Health*, *6*(1), 16–20.

Shufelt, C. (2017). Heart disease in midlife women: True and perceived risk. *Maturitas*, *100*, 106.

Shukla, R., Ganjiwale, J., & Patel, R.(2018). Prevalence of postmenopausal symptoms, its effect on quality of life and coping in rural couple. *Journal of Mid-life Health*, 9 (1), 14–20.

Simon, J. A.,Kokot-Kierepa, M., Goldstein, J., & Nappi,R. E. (2013). Vaginal health in the United States: results from the Vaginal Health Insights, Views & Attitudes survey. *Menopause*, *20*(10), 1043–48.

Stefanopoulou, E., Shah, D., Shah, R., Gupta, P., Sturdee, D. W., & Hunter, M. S. (2014). An International Menopause Society study of Climate, Altitude, Temperature (IMS-CAT) and vasomotor symptoms in urban Indian regions. *Climacteric*, *17*(4), 417–24.

Sternfeld, B., & Dugan, S. (2011). Physical activity and health during the menopausal transition. *Obstetrics and gynecology clinics of North America*, *38*(3), 537–66.

Stong, C. (2012). Menopausal status and ethnicity affect risk factors for stroke. *Neurology Reviews*, *18*(6), 12.

Sun, W. (2017). "The enemy at the door": My friend's lonely and silent battle to breast cancer. In K. M. Williams and F. S. Morant. (Eds.). *Reifying Women's Experiences with Invisible Illness* (pp.123–37). Lanham, MD: Lexington Books.

Sun, W. (2019). A qualitative exploration of Millennial employees' work related stress and retention. In S. Smith (Ed.). *Recruitment, Retention, and Engagement of a Millennial Workforce*. (pp. 103–24). Lanham, MD: Lexington Books.

The American Institution of Stress (2017). https://www.stress.org/.

Tracy, C. S., Dantas, G. C., & Upshur, R. E. (2004). Feasibility of a patient decision aid regarding disclosure of personal health information: qualitative evaluation of the Health Care Information Directive. *BMC medical informatics and decision making*, *4*, 13.

Tsao, L. I., Su, M. C., Hsiao P. J., Gau, Y. M., An, C., & Lin, K. C. (2007). The longitudinal effects of a perimenopausal health education intervention on the mid-life women in Taiwan. *Maturitas*, *57*(3), 296–305.

Vinson, A. H. (2016). Constrained collaboration: Patient empowerment discourse as resource for countervailing power. *Sociology of Health and Illness*, *38*(8), 1364–378.

Wentzer, H. S., & Bygholm,A. (2013) Narratives of empowerment and compliance: Studies of communication in online patient support groups. *International Journal of Medical Informatics*, *82*(12), 386–94.

Westby, C., Burda, A., & Mehta, Z. (2003). Asking the right questions in the right ways: Strategies for ethnographic interviewing. *The ASHA Leader*, 8, 4–17.

White, M. C., Holman, D. M., Boehm, J. E., Peipins, L. A., Grossman, M., & Henley, S. J. (2014). Age and cancer risk: a potentially modifiable relationship. *American Journal of Preventive Medicine*, *46*(3), S7–15.

Woods, N. F. & Mitchell, E. S. (2005). Symptoms during the perimenopause: prevalence, severity, trajectory, and significance in women's lives. *American Journal of Medicine*, *118*(2), 14–24.

Yu, S. M., Huang, Z. J. & Singh, G.K.(2010). Health status and health services access and utilization among Chinese, Filipino, Japanese, Korean, South Asian, and Vietnames chidren in Carlifornia. *American Journal of Public Health*, *100*(5), 823–30.

Chapter Nine

"I like to Read, Play Cribbage, Oh, and I have Alzheimer's"

Managing Interpersonal Relationships and Early Onset Alzheimer's

Jamie Cobb

ROBIN MCINTYRE

Rita Charon wrote in *Narrative Medicine: Honoring the Stories of Illness* (2008), "It is when you are sick that you have to question whom in your life you trust, how much life means to you . . ." (p. 178). Alzheimer's disease, a degenerative brain disease that typically affects older adults, is the most common form of dementia and the sixth leading cause of death in the United States (Alzheimer's Association, 2018). Early-onset or younger-onset Alzheimer's affects people under the age of sixty-five and is often misdiagnosed, hidden behind life stressors. Most people living with early-onset Alzheimer's have sporadic Alzheimer's disease, a form that can affect anyone (Alzheimer's Association, 2018). Robin McIntyre is a vivacious thirty-five-year-old hairstylist who loves to eat, is the middle sister in a family of three girls, is a good friend, likes to travel, and knows how much life means to her. Much like her vibrant personality, Robin is unique. She is part of the 1 percent of the population living with Dominantly Inherited Alzheimer's (Alzheimer Society, 2014). Robin inherited[1] Alzheimer's. Quite unique in experience, Robin's story contributes to the larger body of qualitative research focusing on the patient's perspective of interpersonal relationship and chronic illness management throughout the lifespan. Through a collaborative interviewing and interactive research process approach to narrative inquiry, management of Robin's interpersonal relationships was explored. Relying on theories of social support, communal support, self-disclosure, and illness uncertainty, Robin's story provides a first-hand account of managing interpersonal relationships while living with a chronic illness. This is how her story was collected.

ALZHEIMER'S DISEASE: COLLECTING AND WRITING ROBIN'S NARRATIVE

When Robin was twenty-nine years old, she finally opened the envelope that had been waiting for her for two years. An envelope that her father wished her never to receive. An envelope that too many people in her family have opened, including her mother. Inside this envelope were the results of Robin's genetic screening for Dominantly Inherited Alzheimer's, testing for mutations on the presenilin 1 (PSEN1), presenilin 2 (PSEN2), and the amyloid precursor protein (APP) genes. Mutations on the PSEN1, PSEN2, or APP gene cause overproduction of toxic amyloid-β peptides, causing a build-up of plaques. According to the National Institute of Health, "A buildup of toxic amyloid-β peptide and the formation of amyloid plaques likely lead to the death of neurons and the progressive symptoms of [Alzheimer's]." . . . A person with a mutation on any of these genes is 100 percent certain to have Early-onset Alzheimer's (Alzheimer Society, 2014). Alzheimer's disease is the most common form of dementia and typically affects people over the age of sixty-five, however early-onset Alzheimer's affects those younger. A degenerative disease, Alzheimer's affects the brain through build-up of proteins causing memory loss, inability to carry out normal tasks such as communicating, and eventually it can lead to complete loss of function (Alzheimer's Association, 2014).

Typically, degeneration begins in the memory part of the brain, the hippocampus. Different areas of the brain begin to degenerate as the disease progresses. The U.S. Department of Health and Human Services states, "Memory problems are typically one of the first signs of cognitive impairment related to Alzheimer's" (2018, para. 7). Other symptoms include issues with language and remembering words, as well as issues with vision and spatial awareness (U.S. Department of Health and Human Services, 2018). It is estimated that brain degeneration begins ten or more years before symptoms are present (U.S. Department of Health and Human Services, 2018). People living with Alzheimer's may even experience extreme agitation and even a complete personality change. On average, people living with Alzheimer's live up to ten years following the onset of symptoms. According to the National Institute of Health, "Death usually results from pneumonia, malnutrition, or general body wasting (inanition)" (2018). Currently, Alzheimer's disease, including early-onset Alzheimer's, has predominantly been studied from a medical and physiological perspective in epidemiology, neurology, and other medical fields (see Grøntvedt, Schröder, Sando, White, Bråthen, & Doeller, 2018; Scheltens, Blennow, Breteler, de Strooper, Frisoni, Salloway, & van der Flier, 2016; Cacace, Sleegers, & Van Broeckhoven, 2016). Other scholars have examined the caregiver's perspective providing social support for a family member with Alzheimer's, predominantly focused on the most common type, late-onset (see Baus, Dysart-Gale, & Haven, 2005). Absent from the literature are the narratives of person's living, and coping with, their own Alzheimer's disease. This chapter contributes to the literature on coping with chronic illness throughout the lifespan, primarily focusing on management of relationships and middle-age.

Method

Utilizing a collaborative interviewing and interactive research approach (Laslett & Rapoport, 1975) alongside techniques of narrative inquiry, Robin, in her role as participant, contributed to the primary topics of discussion for the interview guide. The collaborative interviewing and interactive research technique is a process in which the participant and interviewer collaborate through multiple conversations on developing an interview guide to help focus the interview (Laslett & Rapoport, 1975). Throughout the interview, the participant is encouraged to discuss information as their train of thought develops, using the interview guide as a source for direction when a particular topic has been exhausted (Laslett & Rapoport, 1975). Robin's role as co-author also allowed for a self-narrative process to be incorporated. Narrative inquiry focuses on the lived experiences, as told by the people who experience them. Further describing narrative inquiry, Clandinin and Rosiek (as cited in Chase, 2011) argue that everyday experience itself—that taken for granted, immediate, and engrossing daily reality in which we are all continuously immersed—is where narrative inquiry should begin and end" (p. 421). The purpose of narrative inquiry is to collaborate with the participant with the goal of improving their everyday, lived experience. One approach to narrative inquiry is in focusing on how people tell their stories as much as the content of the story (Chase, 2011).

One way to focus on the telling of one's story is to allow them to tell it rather than narrating from a structured set of in-depth interview questions (Chase, 2011). Using collaborative interviewing to develop a guide for the telling of Robin's story, over the span of several months the authors collaborated on the important aspects of Robin's story. Following institutional review board approval to collaborate as co-authors, the first discussion consisted of an overview of the different topics of her story that Robin desired to share and discussed. The second discussion was focused on narrowing down to one particular avenue to focus on her interpersonal relationships. Over the next several months, through several face-to-face meetings, as well as email correspondence, an interview guide was created. The authors met on August 8, 2018, to record the interview. Once the interview was recorded, a transcript was created for analysis and reference purposes. Based on the interview transcripts, the authors then organized the themes that were present throughout the interview. Using these themes as beginning points, and the interview transcript for reference, a narrative of Robin's experiences and interpersonal relationships emerged. This is her story.

Family History

Robin's mother received positive test results in 2006—she carried a mutation. In 2012, at twenty-nine years old, Robin learned her fate; her test came back positive. Although she underwent genetic counseling, and had been through this experience with multiple family members including her mother, it took Robin two years to learn the results of her genetic testing. Robin has never known a life without Alzheimer's. Via autopsy, Robin's maternal great-grandmother was the first in the family confirmed in the 1960s to have Alzheimer's. Robin's grandfather suspected of having Alzheimer's in the 1970s was later confirmed, via autopsy in 1989, to have had Alzheimer's. Robin's mother is one of six children; five of the six carry a mutation including Robin's mother. Robin's uncle Brian, and her uncle Doug, were diagnosed simultaneously in 2004. The next diagnosis came; Robin's mother. In 2013 Robin moved back to the town she considers home to care for her mother. The care her mother needed was taking a toll on Robin's father. Not surprisingly, spouses as caregivers experience a decrease in psychological and physical health, and as the disease progresses, become even more compromised (Martire, Schulz, Helgeson, Small, & Saghafi, 2010). Robin did not want to lose her father also, knowing this disease would eventually claim her mother. Robin's mother passed away in 2016 at the age of fifty-six, still fighting for a cure. Her mother never knew that Robin would be facing the same fate.

Family Is Most Important

Relationships within the family are important throughout the lifespan, and can even continue to have influence long after the passing of a family member. Family relationships not only shape our worldview, they also provide stability and support throughout our lifetime. Afifi and Nussbaum (2006) said, "Families are often the source of our most profound happiness and comfort, and yet they simultaneously function as catalysts of frustration and stress" (p. 276). We often seek the support of our family in the presence of adverse situations, especially when those situations are ongoing. According to Gardner and Cutrona, (2002) family support is so impactful that "Its absence can magnify the damage sustained by adverse life conditions and limit the joy of intimacy with others" (p. 506). Robin's family are experienced; experts even, in support through coping with Alzheimer's. Many of Robin's childhood vacations were spent traveling to the town where her mother grew up, where most of the family remained, for family reunions, funerals, and visits to the nursing home. Robin remembers fondly sharing her first alcoholic beverage with her grandmother during one of the many family trips. She also remembers her grandmother's home as the local hub of socializing. Family were always around, helping each other out, and staying connected through the good times and the bad. There has always been a sense of togetherness. Robin's family even joined the fight for a cure together. At the onset of symptoms in her husband, Robin's aunt began actively searching for research and clinical trials. The family has been actively participating in research since 2004. Few families are plagued with the genetic mutation in such significant numbers of diagnoses, making Robin's family ideal to study. Fortunately, neither of Robin's two sisters have tested positive. Two of her cousins are safe from direct effects of Alzheimer's—their mother (Robin's aunt) does not carry the mutation. Of the remaining eight in their generation, their status is unknown. Despite so much uncertainty of status in the younger generation, each family unit has a unique experience with coping with Alzheimer's, whether it was care giving for a parent or spouse, or providing support for a sibling, aunt, or uncle.

Robin and her two sisters helped their father care for their mother. They know what to expect when the time comes to shift roles from sister to caregiver. Like most siblings, Robin and her sisters have had their share of differences and difficulties. During the oldest sister Jessica's senior year of high school, Robin recalls barely speaking with her. The sisters are certainly talking now. Jessica has agreed to become Robin's primary caregiver when the time comes. The youngest sister has also agreed to help take care of Robin. Both sisters are married and the youngest has children, but they are no less committed to being there for their sister the same way they were for their mother "because that's just what you do for family" (Robin McIntyre, personal communication, August 8, 2018). This is supported in the literature of communal coping. Communal coping is when the collective brings together resources with the shared goal of overcoming difficulties (Afifi & Nussbaum, 2006). This type of coping strategy is particularly useful for managing stress within the family, especially in the context of chronic illness (Afifi & Nussbaum, 2006). Robin's sisters are able to bring together their collective experience as caregivers while providing familial support for Robin when she will need it the most. Jessica is Robin's designated research partner. Each time Robin flies out to participate in research, Jessica goes with her. Robin and her sisters have already begun detailing some of her wishes for when she is under their care. One of these wishes is that dignity must remain intact. This includes hair and make-up. And a therapy dog. She does not want to live to her eighties or nineties. She also does not want to " . . . go out the same way my mom did" (Robin McIntyre, personal communication, August 8, 2018). Despite the years of normal sibling banter, and in preparation for the years to come, Robin and her sisters are extremely close. Their collective experience, and agreement to care for Robin when it's needed, have brought the three closer together. This is something she feels her mother would be extremely proud of.

Until Alzheimer's Do Us Part

Like most twenty-somethings, Robin was navigating life, careers, and relationships. She had dated off and on, eventually investing time into what would become a five-year-long romantic relationship. Throughout this relationship, Robin had managed career changes, living away from home, losing family members, and even her own genetic confirmation. Part of the reason Robin waited the two years between testing and revealing of the results, she did not want the results to influence her life. If there were aspects that she was going to change, she wanted it to be because of a choice, not because of a diagnosis. She and her significant other knew that marriage was most likely off the table for the future; children, however, were still a possibility. As Robin's mother continued her own battle against Alzheimer's, and the test results weighed on her, she realized that this relationship was not sustainable. She wanted something deeper and more meaningful. She was trying to grow in life and he was stuck doing that same thing. While it was a fun relationship, Robin realized as she was planning her future that he was never in it. At times, the social support we seek from others can be damaging to the relationship. A stable relationship is one with balance between input and output (Peterson, 2002). It is expected that as the length of the relationship progresses, understanding of each other's goals, interests, and positions progress (Peterson, 2002). Robin realized he was just not capable of handling "the hard shit" (Robin McIntyre, personal communication, August 8, 2018). At one point toward the end of their relationship, her significant other said he wished Robin had not involved him in anything to do with Alzheimer's. The ending of this relationship was the beginning of another.

Relationships scholars have examined different types of romantic relationships, all the way from erotic relationships to pragmatic relationships (Kelley, 2002). According to Kelley (2002) pragmatic relationships develop as a process of mutual, equitable investment, sustainable through joint admiration and contribution. Pragmatic relationships are often relationships that form over time out of feelings deeper than attraction, in which both persons have interest in relationship investment (Kelley, 2002). Robin's current relationship is certainly pragmatic. During our interview for this chapter Robin said, "he was all in" (Robin McIntyre, personal communication, August 8, 2018). Her current significant other was aware of Robin's family history, as well as the future awaiting her. At one point, before the relationship developed into a romantic one, he told Robin's oldest sister that all he wanted to do was take care of her, even with the Alzheimer's diagnosis. Interestingly, Robin did not have the chance to self-disclose her diagnosis; he already knew. Self-disclosure is important in relationship formation and maintenance, providing opportunity to build trust and closeness (Finkenauer, Kerkhof, & Pronk, 2018). They dated briefly in their mid- to late-twenties breaking up, because even then, he was highly invested in the relationship and Robin was not ready for something quite as serious. The two kept informed on the periphery of each other's lives through friends and family members, with him offering emotional support throughout the different family member's disease progression. When Robin moved home to care for her mom, the relationship began to rekindle. Due to spending more time around each other, and Robin's relationship goals shifting now that she received her diagnosis, both were ready for a more serious relationship.

Robin is still firm in her decision not to have children. More people than in the past are choosing to prolong marriage and children, with some even choosing not to have children at all. However, those choosing to abstain from having children are still in the minority (Afifi & Nussbaum, 2006). Although she does not fault her mother for passing on this disease, she does not want children of her own to go through what she and her sisters went through with their mother. Her current significant other did not have an opportunity for input on this decision. Together they have made other difficult decisions. They go back and forth about marriage, but currently do not see a need. They are focused on buying their house, living life day by day to the fullest, and concentrating on the here and now. Together they live in the moment as much as they can, just trying to enjoy life. As in most secure relationships (Miller, 2015), Robin and her current significant other have mutual interests, such as playing cribbage, eating, and traveling, but they also have their differences. Robin has made a point of trying to say yes to everything. Although she views this as selfish, if something comes up that she wants to do, she is going to do it, whether her significant other is available or not, interested or not. She has traveled by herself and gone on week-long floating trips with complete strangers. She is attempting to live as much life as she can, while she is still able to. She is certain that she has lived more of her life than she has left.

Other Relationships

During one of our conversations in preparation for the interview, Robin mentioned how upsetting it was to watch as some of her mother's friends slowly dwindled out of her life as the disease progressed. Friendships can be just as impactful in our lives as romantic and other family relationships (Blieszner & Ogletree, 2018). Friendship relationships, much like romantic relationships, thrive best when equitable (Ogolsky & Monk, 2018). When we spoke specifically about friendships, Robin said that she knows the friends she's had since early childhood will continue to be there. She also said she has removed people from her life that are "energy suckers" (Robin McIntyre, personal communication, August 8, 2018). She has eliminated people that have caused her grief, hurt her feelings, or have ill intention, because she does not have time for it. There are more important things in her life to worry about. The friendships she developed in early childhood and has maintained, continue to receive her investment and "if anybody else wants to be there, come on in, like, the door's open, but I guess I don't have, I'm not going to output too much because I don't really have a lot to output" (Robin McIntyre, personal communication, August 8, 2018). There are some "on the surface" relationships that Robin has developed, some stemming from her speaking out about Alzheimer's. She feels that some of the people she meets at these events have a need for her to continue to reach out to support them, however her own level of investment is quite low.

One type of relationship that Robin is lacking and desires to have is one of shared experience living with early-onset Alzheimer's. As mentioned above, Robin has a wonderful support system in her family, romantic relationship, and friendships, however she has not had the opportunity to meet a single other person managing early-onset Alzheimer's in the same life stage as her. Her family members were in their forties and fifties by the time they received genetic testing and diagnoses. Her cousins are either negative for the mutation or have not been tested. She knows other people participating in the same clinical drug trial but has yet to meet another person willing to speak up about having the mutation. In this aspect of her illness, Robin feels completely alone.

What the Future Holds

Robin knows that the first person to survive Alzheimer's is out there somewhere, she hopes it will be her. In the meantime, she is actively planning for the worst, while hoping for the best. Part of her strategy is to visualize her brain being healthy. She has no room for self-pity in her fight for a cure. Robin feels it could always be worse. She believes she was given this disease because of her strength to handle it. She hopes to one day attend the weddings of her niece and nephew. Robin is doing things most thirty-five-year-old's are not even thinking about. She has long-term health insurance, life insurance, and a financial planner; things she says most people do in their fifties and sixties. According to Rosato (2018) "over the last five years of life, the average out-of-pocket cost of care for dementia patients totaled 61,500 dollars" (p. 48). Rosato (2018) also states, "With the median household income in the U.S. currently at about $58,000, most people can't remotely afford such a medical hit" (p. 49). She calls her investments risky, but also knows she needs to make money now. If the disease progresses the same way for her as it has for the rest of her family, she knows she will need that financial stability before she is sixty.

Although her future is uncertain, Robin and her family advocate for Alzheimer's research and awareness as the problem and its costs grow. Heid (2018) shows that, Alzheimer's already costs the American health-care system $277 billion annually, and this is a figure that will likely only rapidly increase in the future. Robin and her father frequently speak about their experiences around the nation. She is also participating in research and clinical drug trials. Robin is a firm believer in getting the information out there about Alzheimer's. Over the last several decades, celebrities have come forward and spoken out about Alzheimer's disease and dementia as larger health issue. This list includes Rosa Parks, Gene Wilder, Charlton Heston, and Ronald Reagan (Mifsud, 2018). During his presidency, Ronald Reagan released several statements about Alzheimer's. Following his own diagnosis in 1994, the Ronald and Nancy Reagan Research Institute was created to help fund research (Mifsud, 2018). Despite the heroic efforts of many celebrities advocating for awareness and research, funding is always an issue. Thankfully for Robin and her family, they were able to join a research study, allowing Robin the opportunity to participate in a clinical drug trial. The first year of participation in the clinical trial was rough, taking a toll on Robin as well as her relationship with her current significant other. There were episodes of extreme emotion and constant emotional uneasiness. Robin would go from screaming and being angry to breaking down and crying. She attributes her emotional uneasiness to being scared, as well as the reality of what she is facing. Robin, like many others living with chronic illness, face uncertainties. Mishel's (1988) theory of illness uncertainty explains that illness uncertainty is experienced in four forms: "(a) ambiguity concerning the state of the illness, (b) complexity regarding treatment and system of care, (c) lack of information about the diagnosis and seriousness of the illness, and (d) unpredictability of the course of the disease and prognosis" (p. 225).

Her future in so many ways is uncertain; yet in others, she has first-hand knowledge of what she will be facing. Managing illness uncertainty can be achieved through various means such as seeking information or support. Some researchers suggest that persons living with illness uncertainty wish to maintain their uncertainty since it enables hope (Mishel, 1988). Robin continues to participate in Alzheimer's research as a tribute to her mother and uncles. She also continues to participate knowing this is the only way to find a cure.

CONCLUSION

Robin McIntyre does not know a life without Alzheimer's. When she was young, family vacations were spent visiting her grandfather in the nursing home. He had early-onset Alzheimer's, a degenerative disease that affects people under the age of sixty-five. Not only did her grandfather have early-onset Alzheimer's, he had the rarest form—Dominantly Inherited Alzheimer's. Dominantly Inherited Alzheimer's is a genetic mutation on one of the presenilin 1 (PSEN1), presenilin 2 (PSEN2), or the amyloid precursor protein (APP) genes. A mutation of any of these three genes causes a build-up of plaque in the brain causing degeneration. A mutation is also a 100-percent guarantee of early-onset Alzheimer's. A carrier of the mutation has a fifty-fifty chance of passing on this mutation to each child (Alzheimer's Association, 2018). Robin's grandfather passed on this mutation to five of his six children. One of those five children is Robin's mother. Robin is the middle child of three girls and the only one to have inherited the genetic mutation. Through her journey of care-taking for her mother, receiving her own diagnosis, and joining her family's fight for a cure, she has learned how much life means to her. Supported by theories of interpersonal and family relationship management, Robin's story provides an account of living with chronic illness and managing interpersonal relationships. Robin's story also provides insight into social support, communal coping, and illness uncertainty (Afifi & Nussbaum, 2006; Gardner & Cutrona, 2002; Mishel, 1988). One area left unexplored in this narrative is the management of relationships within the larger family system. Although the purpose of this particular narrative was Robin's management of interpersonal relationships as both a child effected and a patient afflicted by this disease, understanding the relationships of the larger family system would contribute to the existing literature on family communication and chronic illness management. In addition to sharing the lived experienced of interpersonal management and illness uncertainty, Robin's journey has exposed an area for future scholarship. With advancements in genetic testing and understanding of early-onset Alzheimer's, it is becoming increasingly important to understand how persons living with inherited chronic illness cope throughout their lifespan. Further research should also explore how diagnoses, such as Dominantly Inherited Alzheimer's disrupt the lifespan, not just in terms of relationship management, but also in our understanding of the concept of lifespan.

NOTE

1. For more information about Robin's family history with Alzheimer's, see *The Inheritance* by Niki Kapsambelis.

REFERENCES

Afifi, T. D., & Nussbaum, J. (2006). Stress and adaptation theories: Families across the life span. In D. O. Braithwaite & L. A. Baxter (Eds.), *Engaging Theories in Family Communication Multiple Perspectives* (pp. 276–92). Thousand Oaks, CA: Sage.

Alzheimer's Association (2018). Alzheimer's Disease & Dementia. Retrieved from https://www.alz.org/alzheimers_disease_what_is_alzheimers.asp#basics.

Alzheimer Society (2014). Understanding Genetics and Alzheimer's Disease. Retrieved from http://alzheimer.ca/sites/default/files/files/national/research/research_understanding-genetics-and-alzheimers-disease.pdf.

Baus, R., Dysart-Gale, D., & Haven, P. (2005). Caregiving and social support: A twenty-first century challenge for college students. *Communication Quarterly*, 53(2), 125–42. doi:10.1080/01463370500090068.

Blieszner, R. & Ogletree, A.M. (2018). Close relationships in middle and late adulthood. In Vangelisti, A. L. & Perlman, D. (Eds). *The Cambridge Handbook of Personal Relationships* (2nd ed., pp. 148–63). New York: Cambridge.

Cacace, R., Sleegers, K., & Van Broeckhoven, C. (2016). Molecular genetics of early-onset alzheimer's disease revisited. *Alzheimer's & Dementia: The Journal of the Alzheimer's Association*, 12(6), 733–48. doi:10.1016/j.jalz.2016.01.012.

Charon, R. (2008). *Narrative medicine: Honoring the stories of illness.* New York: Oxford Univ. Press.

Chase, S.E. (2011). Narrative inquiry: Still a field in the making. In Denzin, N. K. & Lincoln, Y. S. (Eds.). *The Sage Handbook of Qualitative Research* (4th ed., pp. 421–34). Thousand Oaks, CA: Sage.

Finkenauer, C., Kerkhof, P., & Pronk, T. (2018). Self-disclosure in relationships: Revealing and concealing information about oneself to others. In Vangelisti, A. L. & Perlman, D. (Eds.). *The Cambridge Handbook of Personal Relationships* (2nd ed., pp. 271–82). New York: Cambridge.

Gardner, K. A., & Cutrona, C. E. (2002). Social support communication in families. In Vangelisti, A. L. (Ed). *Handbook of Family Communication* (pp. 495–513). Mahwah, NJ: Lawrence Erlbaum Associates.

Grøntvedt, G. R., Schröder, T. N., Sando, S. B., White, L., Bråthen, G., & Doeller, C. F. (2018). Alzheimer's disease. *Current Biology: CB*, 28(11), R645.

Heid, M. (2018). Breakthroughs in early detection. New techniques make it possible to spot and treat Alzheimer's decades before symptoms appear. *Time, Special Ed.*, 86–90.

Kelley, H. H. (2002). Love and committment. In Kelley, H. H., Bershcheid, E., Christensen, A., Harvey, J. H., Huston, T. L., Levinger, G., McClintock, E., et al. (Eds). *Close Relationships* (pp. 265–315). Clinton Corners, NY: Percheron.

Laslett, B., & Rapoport, R. (1975). Collaborative interviewing and interactive research. *Journal of Marriage and Family*, 37(4), 968–77. doi:10.2307/350846.

Martire, L. M., Schulz, R., Helgeson, V. S., Small, B. J., & Saghafi, E. M. (2010). Review and meta-analysis of couple-oriented interventions for chronic illness. *Annals of Behavioral Medicine*, 40(3), 325–42. doi:10.1007/s12160-010-9216-2.

Mifsud, C. (2018). Stars shining a light. Some celebrated people have helped personalize a disease that's too often shrouded in mystery and secrecy. *Time, Special Ed.*, 70–74.

Miller, R. S. (2015). *Intimate relationships* (7th ed.). New York: McGraw-Hill Education.

Mishel, M. H. (1988). Uncertainty in illness. *Journal of Nursing Scholarship*, 20, 225–32. doi:10.1111/j.1547-5069.1988.tb00082.x.

National Institute of Health. (2018, September 1). Genetics Home Reference. Retrieved from U.S. National Library of Medicine: https://ghr.nlm.nih.gov/gene/PSEN1#conditions.

Ogolsky, B. G. & Monk, J. K. (2018). Maintaining relationships In Vangelisti, A. L. & Perlman, D. (Eds). *The Cambridge Handbook of Personal Relationships* (2nd ed., pp. 523–37). New York: Cambridge.

Peterson, D. R. (2002). Conflict. In Kelley, H. H., Bershcheid, E., Christensen, A., Harvey, J. H., Huston, T. L., Levinger, G., McClintock, E., et al. (Eds). *Close Relationships* (pp. 360–96). Clinton Corners, NY: Percheron.

Rosato, D. (2018). Coping with the costs of dementia: Alzheimer's hits both the mind of the afflicted and the financial security of the entire family. But there are ways to be ready. *Time, Special Ed.,* 48–50.

Scheltens, P., Blennow, K., Monique M. B. Breteler, Strooper, B. D., Frisoni, G. B., Salloway, S., & Wiesje Maria van der Flier. (2016). Alzheimer's disease. *The Lancet*, 388 (10043), 505. doi:10.1016/S0140-6736(15) 01124-1.

U.S. Department of Health and Human Services. (2018). Alzheimer's Disease Fact Sheet. Retrieved from National Institute on Aging: https://www.nia.nih.gov/health/alzheimers-disease-fact-sheet#changes.

Part III

Endings and Legacies

Chapter Ten

Sylvia's Story/The Story of Sylvia

Narrating the Personal and Relational in Patienthood

Leda Cooks

My mother and I have been waiting for almost five hours in a curtained off pre-op room of a local hospital before she undergoes a same day, low risk procedure. Desperate to stay warm in the freezing room, she suggests that we do yoga. We are in warrior pose when the anesthesiologist and nurses enter, and I am asked to leave the curtained pre-op area for five minutes. After ten minutes have gone by, I see a crash cart and multiple doctors running into the area I just left. I can hear loud voices until an attendant shuts the double doors. Then I can hear and see nothing. No one at the desk can tell me what is going on, and no one will let me near my mother's room. An hour and a half later a nurse informs me that sometimes people take a long nap and it is hard for the doctors to wake them up. When I ask her what she means, she repeats the same bizarre explanation. Two hours after that I find out from a "patient liaison" that the anesthesiologist accidentally hit an artery. I am told that my mother bled out, her heart and lungs collapsed, and they had taken her to another part of the hospital where a surgeon had brought her back to life. She is in critical condition—a different surgeon tells me. She might not make it, and I should prepare for this outcome. I call my brother and husband and tell them to get the next flight possible. I call my father, who is in frail health himself and rarely leaves the house and tell him he should try to come to the hospital, a thirty-minute drive. When he arrives, we are taken to the family waiting room, a place I have since come to know quite intimately but which, that day, seems itself a kind of purgatory: a dis/placed space where the usually private expressions of anxiety of families and friends was on display. In the evening, I am informed that my mother's thoracic surgeon (Dr. A) had performed a sternotomy[1] to keep her alive. Now stable, she had lost a great deal of blood. The surgery had been very intense. Her condition was still very uncertain.

Overjoyed at the news she was alive, I had no idea of the degree to which my mother's life and the lives of those closest to her would be altered because of this accident. One of the nurses who had seen my mother before the accident happened, came to visit my mother each day when she was in the ICU. She told the ICU nurses that my mother was amazingly strong, that she had been doing yoga minutes before the procedure was to take place. Over the course of a difficult and tenuous stay in the ICU they called Mom the "yoga" lady. We all told stories about how healthy and active she had been and would be again. Three major surgeries and recurring infections resulting in many long hospitals stays later, my mother's story of who she is and was is constantly changing. What follows is my attempt to better understand my mother's health and healing in relation to the narratives of family, healthcare workers, and caregivers. Central to this inquiry are the questions of how the self shapes discourses and performances of identity, and how others tell stories of life before and after medical trauma. How does the story of who we are as a person merge with stories of patienthood, and how might that change over time and space?

Trauma happens and lives, and life stories, can change overnight. What stories do we tell about who we are now in a present/presence that begs the deconstruction of our past in the telling? Narrative theorists (Fisher, 1984; Ricoeur [see Wood, 1991]) believe that humans are symbolic creatures, and use stories to survive, to order our world through language and chronology. Köber, Schmiedek, and Habermas (2015) observe that, especially among the elderly, "to be understood regarding certain reactions, actions, or characteristics, one may refer to one's life story" (p. 260). Correspondingly, the recognition by significant others of that story becomes increasingly important for healthcare, among other reasons that contribute to quality of life (Hjaltadottir & Gustafsdotir, 2007; Iden, Ruths, & Hjørleiffson, 2015). When life-changing and traumatic events occur across the lifespan, people who are close to us, such as family members, as well as different demographic and social factors, influence the ways we story ourselves in relation to others.

Accordingly, this chapter assumes a relational approach to health communication that considers the construction of patienthood as social and contextual: a negotiation of personhood among caregivers, patients, friends, and family and the spaces in which they interact. Relational approaches to communication pay attention to how power flows in interaction, in the meanings made of conversations and their consequences (Condit, 2006). Rather than document the relative stability or change in my mother's life story after one of several struggles with illness (including two rounds with cancer), or the various interpersonal, social, cultural, and ideological factors at play, in this chapter I examine the ways that different stories about my mother-as-patient are in *tension* or *accordance* with each other as we each work for coherence in our conversations about my mother's health. Any narrative approach relational or otherwise, is ultimately told/written by the author and read through an infinite number of perspectives (Fisher, 1984). However, it is my intention to try to situate stories of who my mother was and is as they became entangled in stories about patienthood—a symbolic rendering of our performances as family and healthcare workers, our relationships, discourses, and actions as they interconnected to make meaning of my mother's health.

This chapter puts my own attempts to narrate my mother's experience in conversation with her stories of who she was and how she sees herself now. I insert my voice in relation to my mother's, both as my stories of self are shaped in relation to hers, and as they connect to those of the doctors, family, and caregivers with whom we are in constant contact. Interspersed throughout the chapter are excerpts from notes taken after visits with doctors inside the hospital and in their offices, conversation and email with my mother, and my own rendering of events. All conversations with healthcare workers indicated in the chapter have been re-created and identifying information of hospitals and caregivers has been altered. These interactions and stories are interwoven with gerontological and communication research on health, narrative, and lifespan identity development. In the last portion of the chapter, I revisit my mother's story in relation to other narratives put forward throughout the chapter. I call for more relational approaches to lifespan health communication that prioritize *how* meanings are made among people in relation to each other, rather than *what* is the content of their message. In the case of Sylvia's (my mother's) story of her life then and now, acquiring a full picture of her health over her lifespan matters less than how she and others narrate the present moment as her past and future as a person and as a patient, as she attempts to recover from a traumatic accident and the intensive surgeries that followed.

SYLVIA'S STORY/THE STORY OF SYLVIA

Four days after the anesthesiologist hit her artery, my mother is slowly coming out of the medical coma. She seems uncertain of where she is. As her eyes fall on me, my brother, and my husband, she tries to smile but then becomes aware of the tube jammed down her throat and grows alarmed. The nurse gives her more sedative and she falls asleep. Because of her panic, we had told the nurses to please wait to tell her what happened—that she in fact was not coming out of anesthesia from the transcatheter aortic valve replacement (TAVR) procedure[2] she had gone in for—that she indeed had never had that procedure and had been in critical condition in the ICU for days. We felt that telling her the truth at this moment would depress and anger her and potentially interfere with her recovery. However, when we return to my mother's room a couple hours later, the nurse tells us that the surgeon had already told my mother what had happened.

Throughout her stay in the ICU, the surgeon will tell his story of my mother many times: to her, to us, and to the medical students who trail him to her room each day. In his story, he is the hero. He has saved my mother's life, he constantly reminds us. He jokes with the medical students that he knows my mother's chest more intimately than anyone. My mother does not find this funny, and I am appalled and offended at his sexism, but since he may be operating on my mother in the future, I do not tell him so.

Older people in the United States are often stereotyped to have diminished mental capacity, low productivity, and general dissatisfaction with life (Nussbaum, Thompson, & Robinson, 1989). These assumptions can be reflected back to them in their everyday interactions when others speak to them as if they are children, speak with raised voices, or assume they are not interested in current events, or do not involve them in significant decision making (Harwood, Giles, and Ryan, 1995). In a narrative review of research on physician perceptions of their elderly patients, Meisner (2012) notes that a significant number of physicians hold negative attitudes about their older patients and prefer not to work with them, although these attitudes vary based on physician age, patient condition, and location (hospital, office, nursing facility, etc.). Worth noting, too, is that as people age and lose status in U.S. society, they must interact more with younger medical workers, new medical knowledge, and new technologies to assist them with healthcare. The amount of new and sometimes contradictory or confusing information they may receive is oftentimes overwhelming, and may be delivered quickly without checking to see if the patient or caregiver has questions (Bergstrom & Nussbaum, 1996). Getting the information and assistance older patients need is often complicated by physicians and surgeons who believe degrading stereotypes, despite prior knowledge of their patient or the patient's actual abilities (Meisner, 2012). For older adults with chronic diseases, such as heart conditions or cancer, both of which my mother continues to battle, continuing to shape one's own story apart from those of health-care specialists is difficult. My mother's ability to give voice to her own concerns and to express potentially competing or alternative perspectives on health and healing was constantly in/formed in relation to others' performances of her treatment.

> Doctor A: We did a thoracotomy and a pneumonectomy.[3] We've pleuridized[4] you so you're dried out. So, let's talk about your AS.[5] I think it's important we go ahead with the heart valve procedure . . .

Sylvia: Before all of this happened, I was told I was the perfect candidate. A lot has changed since then. I've lost a tremendous amount of weight. I'm very weak. It's been five weeks, and I don't feel like I am recovered enough to . . .

Daughter: I understand that you think it is important to move ahead with the procedure, but I don't think you understand what we've been trying to tell you. My mother has been traumatized by what has happened to her. Even discussing this right now causes panic. She needs time.

In this, and many other conversations with us, Dr. A spoke consistently in highly specific medical jargon that we constantly asked him to explain, made eye contact only with my brother or me while verbally addressing my mother, and told us repeatedly that he had saved my mother's life. He told us that because he had performed the sternotomy that saved her, he would do whatever it took to make sure my mother's arteriostenosis would be addressed. For this surgeon, my mother was an investment of effort, skill, and technology. Because the investment was big, he needed to protect it with further surgery. He neither seemed to see nor hear my mother's obvious alarm at the prospect of going back into a risky procedure after almost losing her life. Her subjectivity did not factor into his plans, rather, she seemed to be the object of his projected narrative of heroic success. Meisner (2012), summarizing research on healthcare workers' perceptions of older patients, observes that surgeons, perhaps due to time pressures and the need for quick outcomes, are the least likely of healthcare workers studied to have the time to listen to their older adult patients and most likely to have preconceived ideas of patients' abilities to accurately communicate their problems.

Gerontology research on communication in healthcare facilities (e.g., nursing homes, hospitals), as well as staff and patient interactions, has generally found: (1) little interaction in general (Gaugler, 2014); (2) a predominance of instrumental communication on the part of staff (Bergstrom & Nussbaum, 1996; Mathie et al., 2012); which is based on (3) stereotypes (e.g., speaking as if to a child) and overaccommodative styles (Williams & Nussbaum, 2001); (4) lack of voice or sense of agency among elderly in healthcare contexts (Nussbaum & Coupland, 2004, for exception for males see Seale and Charteris-Black 2008); resulting in (5) dwindling social support and networks (Hagedoorn et al., 2017); leading to (6) diagnoses of depression and overmedicalization for most clients in nursing care facilities, often with little to no interaction (other than task oriented) with the patient (Mathie et al, 2012). Hospital and clinical visits may prove frustrating to both doctors and their older adult patients for several reasons based on time pressure, doctors' expectations regarding patients asking questions if they are confused or concerned, and older patients' assumption that doctors will tell them what they must do (Fisher & Canzona, 2014). However, when older patients do assert themselves they are often equally frustrated by perceived disrespect, and/or short, confusing, or otherwise unsatisfying responses. Although studies of self-care and caretaking at home have shown better overall health for older patients who transition to their home, interactions with healthcare workers continue to play a vital role, not only in effective care, but maintaining quality of life (Bohlmeijer et al., 2011; Fisher & Nussbaum, 2012; Hagedoorn et al., 2017).

COMMUNICATING CARE AND/AS IDENTITY

In view of the focus of this chapter on my mother in relation to others, I want to provide a brief acknowledgment of the context in which caregiving was provided by my brother and me. Like most family histories, ours is much more complicated than is represented here. My brother and I are very connected to our mother, though we live in different parts of the United States, far from the place where we were born and raised. We each have busy lives, with our own families and with full-time jobs. Despite our many attempts to convince our parents to adjust their living arrangements as they have aged, our parents still live independently without a support network of friends or relatives. After the initial trauma set off a chain of reactions that required intensive in-home care, my brother and I worked in overlapping shifts to fly back and forth to care for our mother while maintaining our life and jobs at home. Because of the greater financial loss my brother would endure by (temporarily) relocating to care for my mother, I eventually took over most of the on-site responsibilities for my mother's (and father's) care. From long distance, my brother helped to contact and coordinate her many doctors, and to argue with the insurance agencies over coverage.

Bevan and Sparks (2011) observe that long-distance caregivers become the primary caregivers when this is the only option. My father is a very difficult person, and his bad temperament has been magnified as he grows older and his mobility is limited. His refusal of intensive in-home support (for financial and personal reasons) put the burden on my brother and me to take over nursing responsibilities for which neither of us had been trained or prepared. Soliz and Fowler (2014), in a discussion of the sandwich generation and parent-child roles in middle age, note that middle-aged children most often react to the urgent need for parental care, rather than effectively plan with parents for potential care needs and living arrangements in advance. After years of trying to have proactive planning conversations with our parents, and my father's refusal to consider alternatives, my brother and I each found ourselves in emergency mode, reacting from afar to plan around work schedules and our own family's needs.

Caregiving for a family member, whether due to chronic illness and/or after a traumatic event entails constant assistance with proximal physical needs, such as checking vitals, help with eating, drinking, bathing, providing food and medication, shopping, and washing clothes. Support for emotional needs such as companionship is also required. Both proximal and long-distance caregiving also involves indirect tasks such as negotiations with healthcare providers and outside health service providers, financial management, insurance, healthcare costs, among others (Beekman, 1991; Bevan & Sparks, 2012). In their summary of the research on long-distance caregiving, Bevan and Sparks (2011) discuss the difficulties and anxieties such care presents for caregivers, including deterioration of physical health, increased depression and anxiety, as well as the pervasive feeling among long-distance caregivers that they cannot provide the support needed. My mother's panic attacks and the constant build-up of fluid in her lungs would leave her feeling vulnerable and alone, especially at night, and she would ask that I stay with her. I would sit on the edge of her bed all night, afraid that if I slept she would stop breathing. Although the research indicates negative impacts on health for long-distance (and even more so for long-term) caregivers. This research does not express the liminality I often felt in shuttling back and forth constantly over disparate professional and personal contexts and lives, and the anxiety I experienced, whether at my home and work or with my mother, over her ability to fight for her life and my role in her survival.

Perhaps justifying these anxieties, one morning I heard a crash as I was going to the bathroom and found my mother unconscious on the tile floor in her bathroom. She had landed face down and tangled up in the walker she had had to use since the accident, with its metal bar hitting exactly where the sutures lay over her heart. I called 911. She was taken to the same hospital where the initial botched surgery had taken place. A CAT scan taken shortly after arrival revealed that a radiologist at this hospital had punctured her vein during a thoracentesis[6] two days before. Blood filled her lungs, and her left lung had again collapsed. Again, too, the damage was severe, and the surgery was to be intensive. This time I had to fly home right before the surgery was to take place. In the moments before she was to be taken to the OR, I stood at her bedside with Dr. A. I said goodbye to my mother and told her that I would see her in a few days, after the surgery. Looking terrified, my mother refused to say goodbye to me, telling me she could not leave me. I knew her condition was critical, and the surgery would be difficult, but I left for the airport.

Sylvia, a couple weeks after her second major surgery, speaking to Dr. A in his office:

> I have become a different person. I never had panic attacks before this happened. In fact, I did not know that that is what it is called until someone at the hospital told me that that is what has been happening to me. I never used to be this way. I cannot let my daughter out of my sight without panicking. She needs to be able to leave the house, even to run errands for me, but if she is gone for more than a few minutes I get very anxious.
>
> Doctor: This is fairly common among open-heart surgery patients. I can prescribe anti-anxiety medication but it will take a few months to kick in. Are you taking Xanax? Have you seen a psychiatrist?
>
> Daughter: Her insurance refuses to cover mental health costs. We have tried everything, but the drugs do not reduce the panic attacks. When I do leave the house, she calls and tells me I have to come home because her blood pressure is too high, or she is in terrible pain. I have to be able to leave—to shop, to get her medicine, and for my own sanity—or I will not be able to take care of her.

Common in caretaking situations, my mother and I had shifted in our relationship to each other as she had become increasingly dependent on my support (Beekman, 1991). Nonetheless, after months of anxiety over her tenuous condition, the stress of constant worry and care, and the need to manage my job and family elsewhere, I realized that my mother and I needed to at least take control of the stories we told about who we were in relation to each other. My brother had also come to a similar conclusion, which was revealed in our discussions of how we might work together to continue to care for her. We discussed what the costs of that care might be, financially and physically, as well as to our relationships with family and friends. Bevan and Sparks (2011) observe that family dynamics change, sometimes drastically, when a parent needs care. When parents and siblings live far apart, siblings may communicate more frequently based on the need to discuss the parent's care. My brother and I had gone from speaking once every few months to speaking and texting with each other multiple times a day, discussing my mother's care and the difficulties of life with our father. We both agreed that, in her prolonged patienthood, our fiercely optimistic and independent mother had increasingly become dependent on our care. My brother, also an optimist, strongly believed that if we acted as if she was her old "self," she would begin to rely on us less for emotional and physical support. Because I was around her much more than he was during panic attacks, and doing more of the cooking and cleaning, I found it more difficult to treat her as the mother I had previously instead of our fragile patient in constant need of care.

COMMUNICATING AGENCY

Studying the ways people communicate about life-changing events toward the end of life is less a matter of establishing facticity than it is about understanding how they talk about the events in relation to other traumas they have experienced over their lifetime, the contexts in which they talk, the people with whom they talk, and the various ways power flows throughout their interactions. Communication scholars researching health and aging have studied these interactions interpersonally (Nussbaum, Baringer, Fisher, & Kundrat, 2008), intergenerationally (Barker, Giles, & Harwood, 2004; Williams & Harwood, 2004), and culturally (Pecchioni, Ota, & Sparks, 2004); in terms of communicative competence (Fowler, Fisher, & Pitts, 2014), social networks (Nussbaum & Fisher, 2011), long-distance caregiving (Bevan & Sparks, 2011) and health literacy (Thompson, Parrott, & Nussbaum, 2011), among other areas. Nussbaum et al. state that "[e]ffective communication between the interdisciplinary team, the older patient, and family, friends and caregivers is a necessity" (2003, p. 191). Fisher and Canzona (2014) call for more lifespan communication studies to address the various ways affordances and constraints are created in the multiple contexts of care *for* our elders.

If life storying is an active process (albeit with varying degrees of stability) of interpreting, integrating, and ordering experiences and contexts, (McAdams, 2013), a lifespan narrative perspective is particularly important to qualitative understandings of aging (Webster, 1999). Yamada (2011) differentiates this perspective from "fundamental concepts of developmental psychology and lifespan developmental psychology [that] are both based on assumptions of individualism, the linear progression of life, the privileged status of quantitative measurement, and the irreversibility of time" (p. 420). Lifespan identity development has been characterized as cyclical, with alternating periods of stability and exploration/achievement/transition (Marcia, 1980). Narrative researchers studying identity development later in life differentiate among phases of commitment to stories of the self that stress values, behaviors that allow for continuity, and stories of flexibility and adaption to change (Westerhof, 2009). Antonovsky (1979) also discusses a sense of coherence (SOC) in life narratives; older persons with a weaker sense of coherence tend to suffer more from depression after long-term illness or other mental and physical difficulties, while those with a stronger SOC are more resilient (Westerhof, 2009).

Narrative foreclosure is a concept invoked by some gerontology researchers to describe the narratives of self expressed by older people that are embedded in the past, not open to any new possibilities, and that close off alternative meanings or stories of the self. Bohlmeijer et al. (2011) note that foreclosure may be present at transitional moments, such as declining health, when a senior person might begin to question the stability of life stories. Indeed, such moments may facilitate regrets and challenge stories of a healthy and vibrant self. How older people negotiate these moments is influenced by a number of factors, including the stories of caregivers, family members, friends, and others of significance in their life. Where family caregivers are available and willing they can further support narrative continuity and coherence. Research on family caregiving has shown a positive correlation between supportive family care and better self-care among chronically ill older patients. However, qualitative analysis of planned interactions among medical staff, family caregivers, and elderly patients has shown that, to maintain continuity of care, staff members need more information on the details of caregiving, its contexts, and relationships (Hagedoorn et al., 2017). Transitions in health lead to transitions in stories about a life and the direction of that life story. The ways subjectivity is narrated may be both coherent with one's past and is still always shaped in and by interaction, by communication.

> Daughter: We seem to talk about all this as before and after what happened on October 4. Tell me about what your life was like before and after.
>
> Sylvia: I have always thought of myself as a healthy and active woman. I did not really ever see myself as a patient until all this happened. Even with the cancer and losing all my hair, and then leukemia, which is an ongoing battle, and all of the other surgeries. I always seem to heal quickly so I was focused on getting better. And I have. It seems that everything that happened to me in the past year has stemmed from this one incident. I made the decision to have this procedure because, although I felt fine, I was told that I would feel better after it was done. I did a good deal of research and spoke to friends who told me that they felt better after they had it done, and you told me that story about Jack doing so much better afterward.
>
> But really, I have always been healthy. I have taken care of myself. My whole life I think I have been focused on nutrition. That's something I think I've gotten from my mother. She never ate sugar or processed food, she always believed in vitamins . . . and I've always been active. I was rollerblading in my seventies, and have kept up with the gym and doing yoga. I have always loved art, and the opera. I've been a docent for twenty years, mostly at the Modern Art Museum, but also at the Fine Arts, and the Contemporary Arts Museum. I was still working at the Contemporary Arts Museum when I went in for the procedure. I loved to

go to the Met [in 3D at the movie theater] and to the local opera with my friends.

Really, I try very hard not to think about what happened. It's difficult, but I get very upset when I do. It's not just upsetting because of what it did to me, but the toll it is taking on you and your brother.

For my mother, discussing what happened to *her* is difficult to separate from what happened to *us*. Perhaps if it was not me, her daughter, but an outsider asking her to talk about the experience and impact on her life, she could have made that differentiation and boundary between herself and her family. She could have discussed the changes to her body and concerns for her health with more detachment and with the narrative arc of before and after that we overheard occasionally when she was discussing what had happened with healthcare professionals, insurance agents, and friends with whom she was in contact. The degree to which her concern for our well-being is wrapped up in her own may be reflected in her sense that her suffering is the source of our pain.

Narrative geriatric and communication researchers looking at identity stories in healthcare and caregiving contexts have concluded that older patients, regardless of narrative coherence and flexibility, benefit emotionally from opportunities to be recognized, heard, and responded to by caregivers (Bohlmeijer et al., 2011; Hagedoorn et al., 2017). For many, this is the primary form of interaction in their day, and can benefit emotional as well as physical well-being. Iden et al. (2015) note that the older, chronically ill participants in their study, "endeavor to recreate meaning, make sense of their predicament, and maintain agency," (p. 5) and conclude that healthcare workers can support this endeavor.

[Sylvia and brother, meeting for a consultation with a new thoracic surgeon in preparation for the heart valve procedure never (yet) performed.]

Dr. B: How long did it take you to recover from the first surgery?

Brother: She never had time to recover. After the first surgery she developed fluid in her lungs and had to have a couple thoracentises. We found out later that the radiologist hit her vein during the second one and her lungs filled with fluid and collapsed. She had to have an emergency thoracotomy to locate and drain the fluid. So, no, she never had a chance to recover.

Sylvia: I'm a shadow of myself. My husband and children have been helping me.

[Surgeon points to different parts of my mother's torso.]

Dr. B: (pointing) So you had a thoracotomy here and a sternonomy here, and lots of other scars I can't make out. It's incredible that you survived it, and all with aortic stenosis.

Sylvia: I've always been athletic, I've been very active, and now this happened.

Dr. B: I'm sorry all this happened . . .

My mother has repeated the story of this interaction with Dr. B many times. She talks about it as a pivotal moment for her, one in which she felt someone heard her and her trauma, recognized it, and apologized—if not for his own role in the events—for her suffering.

Sylvia: When Dr. B said that to me, I thought, "Finally, someone has apologized." He understood that what I had been through was awful and should never have happened.

Daughter: I thought Dr. A had told you that it never should've happened to you.

Sylvia: No, I would have remembered that, all that man ever did, was tell me how great he was.

The power to define and be defined through perceptions of identity and agency manifests in communication, and changes as a person ages—perhaps most starkly so when the communication has to do with health (Nussbaum & Coupland, 2004). Lifespan health communication researchers emphasize that the ways we perform an un/healthy identity through communicating to others are important to understand because they offer clues as to what memories are important to bring forth in conversation (Nussbaum, 2014). Williams and Nussbaum (2001) argue that communicating about health is important for older people, both because they have more frequent (intergenerational) and wide-ranging interactions with healthcare workers (Barker et al., 2004), and because health is a frequent topic of conversation with friends and family (Fisher & Canzona, 2014).

THE MIRACLE

Sylvia, during a recent, lengthy hospital visit due to sepsis: "Everyone at the hospital says it is a miracle I am alive. They cannot believe anyone could survive all I have been through."

Subject to the anesthesiologist's accident and the resulting two subsequent heart and lung surgeries in a single month, my mother went from a healthy woman undergoing a fairly low risk procedure to a long-term patient in need of intensive care. After being in a medical coma for four days, she learned about what happened. She had never been able to have the scheduled one-day procedure. Bewildered at first by her inability to speak (the intubation had damaged her vocal cords) and constant panic attacks over which she seemingly had no control, she could not make sense of the narratives about her surgery and recovery told by the doctors and family around her. She later told me that at that time she was too confused and weak to do little more than absorb the stories about what happened by doctors and caregivers. As she gradually gained her voice, so too she gained an ability to listen and respond to other's stories about her in a way that allowed her to shape her own before and after story.

Sylvia's story is one that acknowledges the depth of her trauma, one that establishes a clear distance between who she was and who she is now. Although not the healthy, active woman she once was, she does not foreclose the possibility and indeed, for her, the probability that she will be healthy in the future. Her story does not completely break from seeing herself as a survivor and a fighter. As her body weakens daily with some new problem, often related to hospitalization and medications, she continues to view the new challenges she faces as something she must get through to do the things she was doing before all of this happened. She is determined to move past the miracle of survival to living life as fully as she can.

Her continuous emphasis on framing the future as an active and healthy one also shapes our interactions. We use the words "when you do [x]" . . . and never "if." When possible, we make plans to spend time together that does not revolve around her health. While it makes sense to reframe such experiences, the ways in which they cohere, or do not, with life stories are key to the effectiveness of such narrative strategies on improving the quality of a chronically ill patient's life. Nonetheless, it is not merely the coherence of the narrative to earlier life stories, but the way that power/status moves through interactions from healthcare worker to patient to family, as well as the strength and valence of these relationships that shapes stories told of patienthood. Meanings, whether they cohere or gain traction or not, only do so within these dynamics.

> Sylvia, in an email: Nothing special to write, but it is such a lovely day that I thought I would share my good feelings with you. Had a pleasant time with E. We went to the tearoom as I'm still reluctant to brave the problems with the downtown area. I do want to see the new museum. This is the one that I might docent at (when I'm strong enough and if they ever

need docents). It is all American artifacts (which I know little of, but would love to learn about).

I am going to try yoga at the Y Monday, if I can work it around my doctor's appointment, and, if I cannot, I will go for Wed. Of course, I will take it VERY easy. I have heard it is very crowded but I want to give it a chance anyway.

So . . . enough about me. Did you get that chiropractor appointment for your neck and shoulders? See any more bears in your yard?

Your "ice-cream" card still makes me smile.

Love you, miss you.

My story of my mother's life is reflected in my role as narrator, caretaker, and daughter. Although I have not made it explicit, my story has become coherent with my mother's in interactions with healthcare workers and outside caregivers. As I reflect on my notes of doctor's visits, I see the ways I also shaped my mother's dependence by talking for her when I thought she might be confused, weak, or in pain. Although the contingencies in her story of strength may be noted in her dependence on her family for emotional and physical care, I also reflected that dependency by acting as a caretaker who was sometimes too busy to simply sit and be *with* her as a companion. Our stories of her patienthood merge and converge, as do our relationships: my mother has always been a strong and healthy woman, and she remains so in our stories of her before and after. The tensions in these stories are dialectical, moving between the stories of her independence and dependence, health and disease, (im)mobility, serenity and anxiety, improvements and setbacks.

RELATIONAL NARRATIVES: LESSONS FROM SYLVIA'S STORY

Sarvimäki (2015) observes that narrative methods allow participants' stories to be analyzed holistically, categorically, or both. In the context of stories about health among older persons in Scandinavia, Sarvimäki notes that, when telling a story about one incident (e.g., a fall) older people often contextualize the event within a broader life story. Such narratives may be holistically analyzed as transitional moments in the life story. Many social gerontology researchers (e.g., Bohlmeijer et al., 2011; Kober, Schmiedek, & Habermas, 2015) view life story narratives from the standpoint of social psychology and narrative theory, as a re-storying of the past, providing clues to the effectiveness of patient's coping strategies and quality of life. Lifespan and health communication researchers have analyzed healthcare provider-patient interactions with a focus on processes leading to more effective communication (Fisher & Canzona, 2014). With a focus on communication of narratives about my mother's (healthy) self across the lifespan, in this chapter I have put my narrative as author/daughter/caregiver side by side with differing surgeons' reports to us at her bedside, or in their offices. There were many similar reports and conversations with insurance "case workers," billing agencies, caregivers, and lawyers, not included in this chapter. These reports and occasional conversations with doctors and caregivers are ongoing, and pervade my mother's own stories of before and after, as well as her early silence and then increasing confidence in talking about "what happened." In what follows, I offer some thoughts on the differing ways my mother's narrative of patienthood was fashioned relationally, and what similar research on the way patienthood is communicated might offer those wishing to improve the quality of life for older adults in fragile health.

Sylvia's story of herself as a woman who has always been active, healthy, and strong is constantly in tension with the descriptions of her as a patient found in hospital and surgeon records. In the records, she is described as a frail, petite woman who is suffering from a variety of chronic conditions, and that seemed to be who she became. After the anesthesiologist hit her artery and she was in a medical coma for several days, she began to experience fears that some irreparable damage had been done to her body. She feared she would not be told exactly what that damage had been. She did not feel that Dr. A was being honest with her and this was not helped by Dr. A's seeming discomfort with addressing her directly or with eye contact. Dr. A's consistent insistence that he had saved her life twice demonstrated indifference to, or perhaps a refusal to hear, her experience of before and after the damage was done. My mother's own narrative as a woman whose active and healthy life had been derailed by this accident, was recognized by Dr. B. He affirmed her sense of herself as a strong woman by acknowledging that few people could have survived what she had been through. His support of her description of her patienthood also reaffirmed her life story and in that way, she was able to reconcile some of the ruptures to her sense of self.

Hjaltadottir and Gustaffsdotir (2007) summarize what much lifespan health communication and narrative research has found: that caring and competent communication is key to one's quality of life and hope for a healthier future. Yet, such findings are not easily translated into sets of skills to be practiced by healthcare providers. Stories about being a patient told by older people who have been deeply affected by illness can offer a rich tapestry of interlinking dialectics about identity and belonging, autonomy and dependence, individualism/neoliberalism and communal care that are formed, maintained, and changed through interactions with healthcare workers, care providers, and larger institutional and organizational structures that enable and constrain treatment. In addition to more frequent and caring interaction with clients, Dewar and McBride (2017) promote the use of appreciative inquiry in care settings. Appreciative inquiry in healthcare contexts is focused on questions that ask about what is positive about a person's history, how they have drawn on strengths to deal with current circumstances, and how they envision life getting better. Narrative inquiry can complement appreciative inquiry, moving from asking and responding to questions to telling stories about a life that has changed in terms of adaptation, strength, survival, and growth.

Despite the difficulties we faced and still face negotiating the healthcare system, it is important to note that as a middle-class, white, U.S. citizen, my mother could expect that her most urgent medical needs would be attended to expediently and with competence. Indeed, as a family we all expected that my mother would be treated as the legitimate recipient of care that we felt she deserved. I often had to pause in those moments when I was affronted by the lack of respect shown to us by insurance and healthcare institutions to realize that to even have such expectations came from our class (middle) and race (white) privilege. Although we could not send my mother to the best hospital, she had gone to one she felt (now we realize, wrongly) had a good track record with heart procedures. We expected the best surgical team on offer, and was assured (again, perhaps wrongly) that they were ready to come to my mother's aid. Yes, the elderly in U.S. society have less power and are subject to stereotypes, but within this group and the families and friends that may care for them, it is abundantly clear that there are more and less affordances and constraints that greatly impact health, and consequently survival. Narrative and lifespan research on the health stories of older people, their caretakers, and families could be at the forefront of efforts to understand how stories of patienthood and a life well (or poorly) lived are constructed among older people marginalized by race, poverty, or nationality. The complexities of relationships among people, institutions, technologies, objects, and spaces are underrepresented in the stories told by narrative research, and even fewer representations of these complexities in narratives are seen from researchers and participants who are outside of mainstream U.S. society.

Critical and narrative researchers could also further examine how whiteness and white privilege is negotiated interactionally and institutionally as white patients age and the demographics of healthcare providers change. While patient-centered care is now central to the philosophy of most hospitals, little of the research in this area has examined how such care is communicated across differences in culture, language, race, and class. Older patients now more than ever interact with doctors and other healthcare providers who may be from different countries or speak different primary languages than they do. The majority of my mother's many surgeons and doctors are from other countries, and it is perhaps notable that though Dr. A was white and a

U.S. citizen, my mother did not feel listened to or comfortable with him. She much preferred Dr. B, who was Latino, because he seemed to hear her story and recognized her pain and frustration.

And yet, I wonder how much extra labor is required of Dr. B and other healthcare workers lower in rank and status than he to listen, validate, and otherwise provide support to their older patients. White patients who spend most of their time in hospitals, or who live in nursing homes, may spend much of their day interacting with healthcare workers who are from a race, class, or of a nationality different from them. How are perceptions of listening, being heard, and understood shaped in such intercultural interactions? How do these interactions contribute to stories of patienthood and quality of life? While the former question is occasionally a topic for intercultural health communication researchers (e.g., Kreps & Kunimoto, 1994), both questions could be fruitfully explored in narrative and lifespan health communication scholarship. Nussbaum (2007) argues that communication should be central to any scientific (and I would add social scientific) research on quality of life over the lifespan. Nussbaum observes that a variety of factors seem to influence quality of life as we age, such as engagement with life, degree of loss of abilities, and competence in life tasks involved with social maturation. All are factors seen to occur within the individual, though as Nussbaum (2007) avers, all are acquired in and through communication. How, we might ask, is any measure of the quality of life also a measure of the quality of our communication? Relational approaches to the communication of health and quality of life can deepen our understanding of communication by adding the dialogic to the study of the social construction of meaning and/as identity. Similarly, research on the communication of identity and narrative lifespan research on older adult patients can also benefit from scholarship on aging in place (that is, at home rather than in assisted care facilities) that prioritize the voices of older members in the community in relation to others as partners toward a better quality of life for all (Black et al., 2015). Researching all members of communities (or at least across generational, racial, and income) categories as participants in the healthcare of their senior members illustrates the relationality of stories of aging and health and makes connections across narratives that might not otherwise be made when studying only one population grouping.

Another relational approach not attended to in this chapter is central to the new socio-materialist studies of chronic heart failure, caregiving, and patient self-care. McDougall et al. (2018) study self-care and family caregiving, as they exist in social context through actor network theory (Latour, 2005). They view social context as the entanglement of relationships among people, technologies, in which healthcare outcomes are never fixed or determined by particular interventions but constituted through assemblages of relationships. Such an approach to patienthood over the lifespan might tell a more complex and in-depth story about the ways materials and bodies come together in narratives of subjectivity. In my mother's stories with her friends and family of the incorporation of procedures, surgeries, devices, and (in)abilities, are echoes of medical and cultural stories about what does or does not constitute health and quality of a life.

CONCLUSION: THE STORY CONTINUES

As I am concluding this chapter, after a sleepless night negotiating unsuccessfully long distance with my incoherent mother about going to the ER, my father calls 911 and then calls me at 3:30 am. He tells me that she is unconscious, and it is likely the return of sepsis, but he is not physically able to drive to the hospital to follow her to the ER. Calling the hospital repeatedly, I learn very little. So, I make arrangements to go there as soon as I am able and flights permit. Then I call my brother, change my mind, and decide to wait until I can learn about her condition. Now, nearly a year after the medical accident, I am struck by the degree to which my mother has tried to push away from the dependence she has felt, even as she cannot divorce herself from the realities of her physical condition. As a result, too, she has reconciled her story of a healthy and active woman with one of a patient who can also try to advocate for herself, working to be strong and recover her independence. I, too, have tried to be less available as a proximal caregiver. I call daily, and do my best to balance conversation about her health with other mundane concerns of our everyday lives. My mother is (re)creating a space to tell her own story, a project of salvage and imagination, of healing and reconciliation. As she (re)writes Sylvia's story, we endeavor to better understand our subjectivities in relation to each other.

NOTES

1. Operation to get access to the heart by cracking the sternum open.
2. A minimally invasive procedure designed to open a narrowed aortic valve. Doctors insert a catheter in the leg or chest and guide it to the heart. In most cases, this takes one to two hours and requires an overnight stay in the hospital, with patients walking in a day or two (Mayo clinic, Medtronic). A thoracotomy is performed when a surgeon opens up the ribs to get access to the heart and lungs.
3. A thoracotomy is performed when a surgeon opens up the ribs to get access to the heart and lungs.
4. The surgeon and his team have performed a pleurodesis, essentially vacuuming out the lungs.
5. Aortic stenosis: The narrowing of the heart's aortic valve, which may reduce blood flow and cause heart failure.
6. A procedure to remove fluid between lungs and chest wall.

REFERENCES

Antonovsky, A. (1979). Health, stress, and coping. San Francisco: Jossey Bass.
Barker, V., Giles, H., & Harwood, J. (2004). Inter-and Intragroup Perspectives on Intergenerational Communication. In J. F. Nussbaum & J. Coupland (Eds.), LEA's communication series. *Handbook of communication and aging research* (pp. 139–65). Mahwah, NJ, US: Lawrence Erlbaum Associates Publishers.
Beekman, N. (1991). Family caregiving. Eric digest https://eric.ed.gov/?id=ED328826.
Bergstrom, M. J., & Nussbaum, J. F. (1996). Cohort differences in interpersonal conflict: Implications for older patient-provider interaction. *Health Communication, 8,* 233–48.
Bevan, J. L. & Sparks, L. (2011). Review: Communication in the context of long-distance family caregiving: An integrated review and practical applications. *Patient Education and Counseling, 85* (1), 26–30. DOI: 10.1016/j.pec.2010.08.003.
Bevan, J. L., Vreeburg, S. K., Verdugo S., & Sparks, L. Interpersonal conflict and health perceptions in long-distance caregiving relationships. *Journal of Health Communication, 17* (7), 747–61. ISSN: 1081-0730 PMID: 22642716.
Black, K., Dobbs, D., & Young, T. (2015). Aging in Community: Mobilizing a New Paradigm of Older Adults as a Core Social Resource. *Journal of Applied Gerontology, 34* (2), 219–43, DOI: 10.1177/0733464812463984.
Bohlmeijer, E. T., Westerhof, G. J., Randall, W., Tromp, T., & Kenyon, G. (2011). Narrative foreclosure in later life: Preliminary considerations for a new sensitizing concept, *Journal of Aging Studies, 25* (4), 364–70 DOI: 10.1016/j.jaging.2011.01.003.
Condit, C. (2006). Communication as relationality. In G. J. Shepherd, J. St. John & T. Striphas, (Ed.), *Communication as . . . .Perspectives on theory.* (pp. 3–12). Thousand Oaks: Sage.
Dewar, B., & McBride, T. (2017). Developing caring conversations in care homes: An appreciative inquiry, *Health and Social Care in the Community,* 27(4), 1375–386.
Fisher, C. L., & Canzona, M. R. (2014). Health care interactions in older adulthood. In J. F. Nussbaum (ed.), *The Handbook of Lifespan Communication* (387–404). New York: Peter Lang.
Fisher, C. L., & Nussbaum, J. F. (2012). "Linked lives": Mother-adult daughter communication after a breast cancer diagnosis. In F. C. Dickson & L. M. Webb (Eds.), *Communication for families in crisis: Theories, research, strategies* (pp. 179–204). New York: Peter Lang.
Fisher, W. R. (1984). Narration as a human communication paradigm: The case of public moral argument. *Communication Monographs, 51,* 1: 1–22.
Fowler, C., Fisher, C. L., & Pitts, M. (2014). Older adults' evaluations of middle-aged children's attempts to initiate discussion of care needs. *Health Communication, 29,* 717–727.
Gaugler, J. E. (2014). Aging of communities: Communities of aging. *Journal of applied gerontology, 34,* 2: 134–137.
Giles, H., Coupland, N., Coupland, J., & Nussbaum, J. (1992). Inter-generational talk and communication with older people, *International Journal of Aging and Human Development, 34,* 271–94.
Hagedoorn, E. I., Paans, W., Jaarsma, T., Keers, J. C., van de Schans, & M. L. Luttik.(2017), Aspects of family caregiving as addressed in planned discussions between nurses, patients with chronic conditions and family caregivers: A qualitative content analysis, *BMC Nursing,* 16, 37–47.
Harwood, J., Giles, H., & Ryan, E. B. (1995). Aging, communication, and intergroup theory: Social identity and intergenerational communication. In J. F. Nussbaum & J. Coupland (Eds.), LEA's communication series. Handbook of communication and aging research (pp. 133–59). Hillsdale, NJ, US: Lawrence Erlbaum Associates, Inc.
Hjaltadottir, I., & Gustaffsdotir, M. (2007). Quality of life in nursing homes: Perceptions of physically frail elderly residents. *Scandinavian Journal of the Caring Sciences,* 21(1), 48–55.
Iden, K. R., Ruths, S., Hjørleiffson, S. (2015). Residents' perceptions of their own sadness-a Qualitative study Norwegian nursing homes, *BMC Geriatrics, 15,* 21–28.
Kober, C., Schmiedek, F., Habermas, T. (2015). Characterizing lifespan development of three aspects of coherence in life narratives: a cohort-sequential study. *Developmental Psychology,* 51(2), 260–75.

Kreps, G. L. & Kunimoto, E. N. (1994). *Effective communication in multicultural healthcare settings.* Thousand Oaks, CA: Sage.

Latour, B. (2005). *Reassembling the social: An introduction to actor-network theory.* New York: Oxford University Press.

Marcia, J. E. (1980). Identity in adolescence. In J. Adelson (Ed.), *Handbook of adolescent psychology* (pp. 159–87). New York: Wiley.

Mathie, E., Goodman, C., Crang C., Froggatt, K., Iliffe, S., Manthorpe J., et al. (2012). An Uncertain future: The unchanging views of care home residents about living and dying, *Palliative Medicine*, 26 (5), 734–43.

McAdams, D. (2008). Personal narrative and the life story. In John, Robins & Pervin (Eds.), *Handbook of personality: Theory and research.* (pp. 241–61). New York: Guilford Press.

McAdams, D. P., & McLean, K. C. (2013). Narrative identity. *Current directions on psychological science*, 22, 3: 233–238.

McDougall A., Kinsella, E. A., Goldszmidt M., Harkness K., Strachan P., Lingard L. (2018). Beyond the realist turn: A socio-material analysis of heart failure self-care. *Sociology of Health and Illness*, 40(1):218–33. doi: 10.1111/1467-9566.12675.

Meisner, B. A. (2012). Physicians' attitudes toward aging, the aged, and the provision of geriatric care: A systematic narrative review. *Critical Public Health*, 22 (1), 61–72. doi: abs/10.1080/09581596.2010.539592.

Nussbaum, J. F. (2007). Life Span Communication and Quality of Life. *Journal of Communication*, Vol. 57 Issue 1, 1–7. 7p. DOI: 10.1111/j.1460-2466.2006.00325.x.

Nussbaum, J. F. (2014). *Handbook of lifespan communication.* New York: Peter Lang.

Nussbaum, J. F., Baringer, D., Fisher, C. L., & Kundrat, A. (2008). Connecting health, communication, and aging: Cancer communication and older adults. In L. Sparks, H. D. O'Hair, & G. L. Kreps (Eds.), *Cancer, communication, and aging* (pp. 67–76). Cresskill, NJ: Hampton.

Nussbaum, J. F., & Coupland, J. (Eds.). *Handbook of Communication and Aging Research* (2nd ed). Mahwah, NJ: Erlbaum.

Nussbaum, J. F., & Fisher, C. L. (2011). Successful aging and communication wellness: Understanding aging as a process of transition and continuity. In Y. Matsumoto (Ed.), *Faces of aging: The lived experiences of the elderly in Japan* (pp. 263–272). Palo Alto, CA: Stanford University Press.

Nussbaum, J. F., Thompson, T., & Robinson, J. D. (1989). *Communication and aging.* New York: Harper & Row.

Pecchioni, L. I., Ota, H., & Sparks, L. (2004). Cultural issues in communication and aging. In J. F. Nussbaum & J. Coupland (Eds.), *LEA's communication series. Handbook of communication and aging research* (pp. 167–214). Mahwah, NJ: Lawrence Erlbaum Associates Publishers.

Sarvimäki A. (2015). Healthy ageing, narrative method and research ethics. *Scandinavian Journal of Public Health.* 43(16):57–60.

Seale, C., & Chateris-Black, J. (2008). The interaction of age and gender in illness narratives. *Ageing and Society*, 28 (7), 1025–1045. doi:10.1017/S0144686X0800737X.

Soliz, J. & Fowler, C. (2014). Sandwich relationships: Intergenerational communication. In J. F. Nussbaum (ed.), *The Handbook of Lifespan Communication*, (293–310). New York: Peter Lang.

Thompson, T. L., Parrott, R., & Nussbaum, J. F. (2011). (Eds). *The Routledge handbook of health communication* (2nd edition). New York: Routledge.

Webster, J. D. (1999). World views and narrative gerontology: Situating reminiscence behavior within a lifespan perspective. *Journal of Aging Studies*, 13 (1), 29–42. doi: 10.1016/S0890-4065(99)80004-8.

Westerhof, G. J. (2009). Identity construction in the third age: the role of self narrative. In H. Hartung & R. Meirhofer (Eds.), Narratives of lives: mediating age (pp. 55–69). Münster: LIT.

Williams, A. & Nussbaum, J. F. (2001). *Intergenerational communication across the lifespan.* Mahwah, N.J.: Erlbaum.

Wood, D. (1991). (Ed.). *On Paul Ricoeur: Narrative and interpretation.* New York: Routledge.

Yamada, A. (2011). Culture and psychopathology: Foundations, issues, directions. *Journal of pacific rim psychology*, 10: 42–103.

Chapter Eleven

Linked Lives

A Narrative Exploration of Positivity and Dialectic in a Patient's Experience

Deleasa Randall-Griffiths

When Fisher (2011) tells the story of her mother's cancer experience, she emphasizes the intricate mother-daughter connection by titling the chapter "Her Pain Was My Pain" (p. 57). Fisher's perspective of a "shared mother-daughter health crisis" (p. 59) mirrors my connection to my mother's health journey. Fisher (2011) writes of the dialectical role reversal set forth when illness strikes, when a daughter shifts into the role of caretaker for the woman who, for years, has taken care of her. As my mother's health declined near the end of her life, my need to nurture her, to work as a team, placed me in the both/and of a daughter mothering her own mother. Fisher (2011) reports that just "being there" is a key theme of support and care during a mother-daughter health crisis (p. 60). I write this mother-daughter story in hopes that those reading will connect it to their own story of shared joy and pain. It is a story about my mother's positivity and her ability to navigate dialectic tensions on the final stages of her personal health journey.

"Humans are creatures of story, so story touches nearly every aspect of our lives" (Gottschall, 2012, p. 15). What we experience in life comes to us in fragments, fractured and in disarray. What story allows us to do is make it whole. Birch and Heckler (1996) suggest looking at stories with the metaphor of nets used by hunters to carry away their bounty. Similarly, we carry away the bounty of our life experiences in a "spirit net" filled with stories. Just as the net retains only the larger chunks of meat from the kill, so do our stories retain the larger chunks of memory, capturing the essence, but leaving behind less significant details. They also liken stories to "a mental opposable thumb, allowing humans to grasp something in their minds—to turn it around, to view it from many angles, to reshape it" (Birch and Heckler, 1996, p. 11). As one who studies human communication, this manipulation of ideas fascinates me. I believe in the power of sculpting experience into story as our primary means of connection and understanding. Telling this story of my mother's medical events tethers me to her life's journey. It also guides me forward on my own life journey. Shared stories touch more lives than just the individuals involved in the experience. Kellett (2017) points to ways in which hope can be "co-created through talk" by the sharing of health stories. He states, "when people can relate to the information in a way that enables them to share connections to their lives in that moment then it can be a positive dynamic" (p. 48).

POSITIVITY AND POSITIVE COMMUNICATION

Positivity is the overarching theme of my mother's story. For her, this was a fundamental life-choice. There is a picture still hanging on the wall of my Dad's house. It reads: "I get up, I walk, I fall down. Meanwhile I keep dancing." My mother loved these words and they encapsulate how she lived and how she died. Fisher, Miller-Day, and Nussbaum (2013) note that positivity can be evidence of a "philosophy of living" (p. 105). When she was a child, her eight-year-old brother died of lockjaw. He was her playmate and her best friend. Without much choice, she kept dancing. In her middle years, she was a twenty-year survivor of cancer. From that point on she encouraged countless others with a message of hope, healing, and positive thinking. In her last years, she learned to live with a body that was slowly deteriorating, providing her less and less mobility. All the while, she strived to live her life to its fullest. She kept on dancing.

Given the physical challenges she faced for so many years, her optimism and gratitude were an inspiration to everyone who knew her. Sullivan (2013) found that gratitude, humor, and laughter all contribute to the benefits of positive communication on physical, emotional, and relational health. She looked at life not just as a "glass half-full," but as one that overflowed with possibility and hope. She lived her life as an example of how to love, laugh, and live life to its fullest. She kept on dancing, so that others could dance alongside her. At her funeral, I reminded everyone that she would be the first to tell us all to "just keep dancing."

Pitts and Socha saw a need for more research on the impact of positive communication. Their call for scholarly contributions was so successful that they published two books on the subject (Socha and Pitts, 2012; Pitts and Socha, 2013). The second volume focuses specifically on the ways positivity connects to health and wellness. Their collection combines work in positive psychology with communication theory and practice. Research covers a range of benefits positivity can bring to individuals' health and relational wellness. It also examines the influence of positivity on healthy institutions.

Kellett (2017) speaks of positivity as a culturally valued American narrative archetype. While many people focus on the virtues of this pervasive value, others point to the maladaptive side that might invalidate feelings and prevent the expression of negative attitudes (Fisher, Miller-Day, and Nussbaum, 2013). Ehrenreich (2001) was one of the early public critics of the expectation of positivity she experienced during her battle with breast cancer. What she called the "bright siding" of cancer challenged the idea of a direct link between overcoming cancer and maintaining a positive attitude. Still, much research supports the notion of positivity and positive communication as a key component of health.

Fisher, Miller-Day, and Nussbaum (2013) discuss the role of the mother-daughter relationship in the healing process and the importance of a healthy dose of positivity. Much of their findings focus on the adaptive contributions of positivity between mothers and daughter and the reciprocal effect of reframing perceptions from negative to positive. The impact of my mother's positivity extends beyond her life and death. Three years after her death, I wrote the following journal entry.

> As I walked today, I thought of something I have not thought of in all the 8 weeks of daily morning walks. I thought of my Mom. I thought about how she could not walk the entire last year of her life. I thought about how much I take my legs, my back, and walking for granted. She probably did too. But, that last year or so, as she slowly lost the use of her legs, I am sure she did not take it for granted any longer. She didn't talk much about that aspect. She stayed so positive, always focused on what she had, what she could do, not what she could not. That was her style in all of life. That was how she made it through cancer in the mid-90s. That is how she jovially handled the daily hookup to the machine that lifted her from one chair and deposited her onto another. So, that is what I thought about today on my walk. It occurred to me that she is why I must walk. I walk for her, even when she has been gone for 3+ years. I walk today because I can. I walk today because she could not. She is still teaching me lessons about how to live my life.

DIALECTIC TENSIONS

As I look back at the last few years of my mom's life, combing through her meticulously charted health history and matching that to my memories, I see connections to Baxter and Montgomery's (1996, 1998) Relational Dialectics Theory (RDT). In research that predates the formation of RDT as a theory, Miller and Knapp (1986) studied the dialectical communication needs during end-of-life situations. O'Hara (2017) documents several examples of several studies using RDT as a framework to study interpersonal and family relationships with healthcare contexts. Keeley and Generous (2015) look at final conversations from a RDT framework. Similarly, Golden (2010) uses RDT to analyze her personal experiences during the death of her grandmother. She outlines similar sets of dialectical tensions: certainty and uncertainty, control and lack of control, and autonomy and connectedness. Amati and Hannawa (2014, 2015) explore RDT with regard to physician communication with patients and family members during end-of-life situations, noting issues of openness and expression as one of the many relational dialectics impacting communication.

Baxter and Montgomery (1996) write about "'dialogic complexity' or the 'both/and'-ness with respect to the knot of contradictions present at a given point in time" (p. 58). During this time of increasing change, my mother was both patient and practitioner during periods of change and stability. She dealt with shifts in autonomy and connectedness. As her life became a blend of public and private encounters, she exhibited a balance of resilience and fragility. Baxter and Montgomery (1996, 1998) see communication among individuals as the primary means to negotiating these types of contradictions in daily life. That was certainly true for my mother.

BOTH PATIENT AND PRACTITIONER

My mother's orientation to life as a healthcare practitioner came at an early age. Her grandfather practiced medicine as a country doctor in rural Indiana. At the age of fifteen, she was working as a nurse's aide in the local hospital where she met my father. She was an emergency room nurse who eventually left the hospital setting for a career as a county health nurse. Her identity was steeped in the world of nursing. Throughout her life, as she experienced a range of health issues, she always approached them from the perspective of a nurse. Several nurses have written about the role ambiguity of nurses as patients (Cardow, 2017; Celaya, 2018; Edward, Giandinoto, and McFarland, 2017; Knight, 2018). Most describe the experience of being a patient with a similar perspective of insider awareness, while at the same time concluding that their experience as a patient made them a better nurse.

My mom played the role of patient in many of the standard scenarios. She gave birth to four children. She broke her leg twice, had her tonsils and appendix removed, had a full hysterectomy, eventually had both knees replaced, and ended up developing diverticulosis and arthritis in her later years. None of the health issues individually or collectively makes her story unique. She was also a twenty-year survivor of non-Hodgkin's lymphoma, which required both chemo and radiation treatment to her spine.

My mother knew that nurses often make the worst patients. She knew they could be condescending, uncooperative, and demanding as patients. She prided herself in being just the opposite. She was the model patient, always pleasant, compliant, and mindful in her requests for a nurse's time and care. She tried so hard not to be a bother while in the hospital. A few times family members had to step in and advocate on her behalf for the care she needed. She always performed her role as patient within the dialectical boundaries of a healthcare practitioner.

CHANGE VERSUS STABILITY

The dialectic of stability and change is a constant for us all. With health issues, one sometimes only notices periods of stability when punctuated by degeneration and decline. Kellett (2017) notes "how fragile the myth and reality of 'stability' were when set against its dialectic partner—decline—in a degenerative disease path" (p. 5).

Prior to the diagnosis of her cancer in 1993, my mom experienced back pain that resulted in years of treatments. First was the surgical removal of bone spurs from her lumbar in 1990. As her back problems progressed into severe scoliosis, she underwent multiple injections and epidurals and finally another major back surgery in 2002. This operation fused her spine together from the last two thoracic vertebrae all the way down through all of her lumbar vertebrae. Her surgery wounds took weeks to heal and an unexpected seventeen days in the hospital. Doctors were puzzled by the slow progress, but keenly aware that the very radiation treatments that had helped save her life a decade before had also severely damaged the tissue in her spinal region. That surgery kept her mobile for a few more years: but not without assistance and not necessarily pain-free. One hip was significantly higher than the other hip. She wore customized shoes with a two-inch lift on one side. She tried massages for pain, physical therapy, and injections. By 2010, six years after that last surgery, her medical notes are "Last x-rays showed further degeneration in lower back. Walk when shopping with cart. Walk with walker due to back problems. . . . After rehab I was walking with cane but fell. Dr. advised that I stay with walker."

"In matters of health, things tend to change quickly for the worse, and slowly for the better. When they change for the worse, the experience can be disruptive traumatic, shocking, and off-balancing" (Kellett, 2017, p. 21). The first time I realized things were continuing to decline for my mother was on my sister's wedding day in 2012. Mom slipped while getting into her van to go get her hair done. She could not pull herself up and into the vehicle. She could not stand either. Luckily, my husband heard her calls for help and came running. She was desperately hanging on to the steering wheel. Her feet completely gave out on her and she could not get back to a standing position. It was the first real sign that something was very wrong. We watched her closely throughout the outdoor ceremony and reception. She carefully walked over bumpy terrain, with the aid of her walker, to pose for family photos by the lake. After that day, it was easy to ignore the subtle changes.

By the next year, my mom showed further signs of decline. She fell several times, at church and out shopping. Once she fell in the shower and my Dad said, "She was holding on to the grab bars for dear life." Sometime along the way, she bought a motorized scooter for longer walking needs. However, she still used her walker most of the time. My parents had a lift installed in their van to transport the scooter.

What we now know is, her legs were slowly becoming more and more paralyzed and her ability to control them was diminishing. Her medical notes say "Losing use of legs. Tender Care [a local home healthcare provider] to home. Legs getting worse." By spring 2013, she was less and less able to stand/walk. My brother came to the house seven or eight times a day to transfer her from chair to scooter, scooter to toilet and back again. In May 2013, the doctor finally admitted her into the rehab unit of the local hospital. At first, the physical therapists tried to help her walk again, the primary goal of their training. Finally, they realized walking was no longer possible. Neurologists confirmed that scar tissue, now tethered to her spinal cord, made surgery far too risky. That is when we knew we had reached some strange point of no return. There would be no more standing, no more moving from chair to chair, no more walking on her own.

From that point forward, our journey became one of shifting identities. My mother and I never talked about it directly, but the permanence of these changes must have been shocking. Kellett (2017) says, "such a struggle can have us trying to hold onto how things were when we had control, and when things made sense" (p. 21). She must have asked herself questions similar to Kellett's "Who will I become, and what will this mean?" (p. 21).

AUTONOMY AND CONNECTEDNESS

Kellett (2017) calls his loss of vision a "crisis of independence" (p. 33). This aptly describes my mother's experience of losing the use of her legs. She had always been one of the most independent women I knew. She had her own career, took on leadership roles in her community, and lived a very independent life. Suddenly, all of that changed. While she was in rehab, I researched accessibility equipment to compensate for the loss of her legs. We needed a mechanical replacement for my brother who could not continue his daily efforts. The hospital used a machine called the Easy Lift. It was by no means cheap, but of all of the options, it was the best. We purchased the exact same device the hospital used. The machine cost several thousand dollars, but it was the only replacement for my brother, who had patiently moved her multiple times a day during that spring. The Easy Lift had a harness she put around her back and under her arms. It buckled on her like the ski belt I have seen used at the lake. Once attached with her feet placed on the platform, the lift automatically assisted her up to an almost-fully-standing position. After that, someone could roll the unit, transporting her from place to place. It struck me as a bizarre and tragic amusement park-like ride.

We assessed other mobility needs for the future. My parents bought a used power wheelchair and a used ramp van to transport my mom. Their house needed several renovations done quickly. The wheels of the Easy Lift did not work well on carpet. Since my aging father would be doing most of the daily transporting back and forth from bedroom to kitchen, kitchen to bathroom, bathroom to living room, and on and on . . . we needed to make things as easy as possible. Luckily, my brother could quickly rip up carpet and install laminate flooring.

During the renovations, I emptied bookcases and china cabinets full of family heirlooms. My mom told family stories that went with each item. I listened intently, trying to hold on to as much of her wisdom as I could. We decided to label the items as we went. The unspoken truth we both knew was that someday she would no longer be present to tell the stories. In the midst of all the changes and upheaval, my mother took advantage of an opportunity to connect me with the past, our family's past. It was another example of her positive attitude. Instead of wallowing in self-pity, she focused on the stories she could share with me.

We replaced my parents' queen sized bed with a rented hospital bed. It had a special inflatable air mattress specifically designed to prevent bedsores. My mom used one similar to it while in rehab. The rental unit was more rustic, but we hoped it would suffice. My dad now slept next to her in my nephew's old twin bed. Mom told me he had kissed her goodnight every night of their married life. That kiss had to make its way across side rails, but the ritual continued each night.

PUBLIC VERSUS PRIVATE ENCOUNTERS

We put a baby monitor in my parent's bathroom. It was the only bathroom large enough to accommodate the Easy Lift. However, it was far from the main parts of the house. The monitor gave my mom a way to signal when she was done and needed someone to come and get her. Unfortunately, it also amplified any bathroom sounds. We tried to remember to turn the volume down when others came to the house. The entire set up backfired at times and she would remain stranded with no one hearing her calls. There were no easy answers. This was one of the many ways she lost her privacy along with the use of her legs. Nevertheless, she kept her positive attitude most of the time. She rarely complained about all the ways her private life had become public display.

We tried our hardest to make accommodations, but still keep things as close to normal as we could. In fact, the abnormal ways of life, hoisting my mom on the Easy Lift and pushing the lift from room to room with her body dangling from its harness in a half crouch/half standing position all became normal. Positioning her above the toilet and then pulling down her pants before I eased the lift down became commonplace. She could handle all of her own personal care needs. As long as we brought her clothing and supplies, she was very self-sufficient. I learned that a person could accomplish all manner of activities, including bathing and getting dressed, from the seat of a toilet.

A variety of home health workers, nurses, occupational therapists, and physical therapists, came to the house. Some were less than satisfying in their bedside manner and care. Most were very knowledgeable, kind, and caring. They became like friends. They came in and out of the house, dressing her bedsores, teaching her to accommodate for her loss of mobility, and trying to keep as much strength in her legs a possible, which was still needed to stand on the Easy Lift.

Mom developed severe wounds on her rear end from sitting too much. We bought every kind of chair pad you can imagine trying to prevent this from happening. She spent most of the summer on twenty-hours-a-day bedrest because she developed bedsores that would not heal. She had weekly appointments at a hospital Wound Care unit. These visits must have been so awkward and uncomfortable. Nurses and aids would hoist her up on an examining table. She would lay on her side on a hard table, her backside covered only with a thin sheet. The wait to see a doctor lasted over an hour sometimes. Each week we learned that the wound was not healing yet. More bedrest, more appointments, became the standard directive. My parents and sister spent their summer going back and forth to these weekly appointments. Crammed in a tiny room, not meant for comfort, they waited patiently. I have heard my sister say many times, she hated those appointments, but looking back, she would give anything to have even that time with my mom back again.

As summer turned to fall, the changes became commonplace. We settled into new routines that included group effort to accomplish the simplest daily tasks. In September, we hosted an eighty-third birthday party for my mom and invited family and friends. There was laughter and celebration throughout my parent's house that day. Memories of "the good old days" were in the air, even as my mother drove her power chair from room to room visiting with guests. However, there were moments where our bizarre daily routines, now normalized from their frequency, interrupted the gaiety. One example was when I harnessed my mom to the Easy Lift, an act I had performed dozens, if not hundreds of times, and began pushing her past the guests on the way to the bathroom. There was an awkward silence in the room and looks of discomfort and concern on people's faces. My mother and I both just smiled and carried on as if nothing out of the ordinary had occurred. For us that was true. For these loved ones, still getting used to the reality of my mom's daily existence, there was nothing ordinary about the Easy Lift.

I came for frequent visits, taking over all the assistive duties in order to give my dad a break. The strain of moving the Easy Lift was wearing on him, I could tell. He never said a word to me, but my mom told me his wrists were bothering him. The average day had a complex routine that required multiple exchanges and movement around my parent's spacious house. We moved my mom from bed to toilet, toilet to power chair for breakfast time, power chair back to toilet for daily personal care and dressing for the day, and toilet to recliner in the living room for reading and TV. As my mother lost feeling, she also lost her ability to perceive bathroom needs. We followed an every-three-hours plan to prevent incontinence. The nighttime routine included a "tucking in" reminiscent of childhood. I would lower my mother on to her hospital bed and gently lift her legs, positioning her on the bed. I would remove her shoes, tuck in the blankets, and softly kiss her goodnight. She welcomed the affection and warmth. She frequently expressed gratitude for all my assistance.

That Christmas, I introduced my mother to online shopping. She became an instant fan. It was one of the ways I tried to reconnect her to her old life. She had always been an avid shopper. In terms of mother-daughter activities, it was top of the list. I created mailing labels for her Christmas cards and printed off copies of a hand written letter she included with each card. She playfully shared the changes of the past year. As always, she kept the mood light and the message positive. The last line of the letter read "I am learning there is life without legs." Reading Scholl's (2013) research on humor as a tool for coping with illness validated my mother's positivity choices.

RESILIENCE AND FRAGILITY

In their analysis of interviews with nurses who returned to work after dealing with cancer, Edwards, Giandinoto, and McFarland (2017) found being resilient as one of the common themes. They note "humour, spirituality, and positive affirmations" as common strategies for resilience (p. 1173).

According to my mom's April calendar, life was moving along smoothly. She marked "good check-up" by her oncologist visit. She kept weekly appointments to get her hair done, had lunches out with friends, and played cards with my aunts and uncles. We enjoyed a lovely Easter visit. On the days in between events, she wrote "Rest." She was moving more slowly, but she was still active and engaged. My parents celebrated their sixty-second wedding anniversary on April 13. Toward the end of the month, my parents attended a reunion at the outpatient rehab unit. Mom wrote "great time" in her calendar that day.

Friday, May 2, I received a call that Mom was admitted to the hospital. She had cancelled her Friday hair appointment, going instead to see her doctor because of shortness of breath. They admitted her right away, thinking it was lung related. I drove to town late that night and went to see her the next day. I noticed the room she was in was much larger than a normal hospital room. It had a couch at the far end and lots of extra space. The staff told her it was their hospice room. If no one was using it and the wing was full, they could utilize it to quickly admit a new patient.

May 3 in my mom's calendar notes "Heart Problems." This was the first time we heard that she had heart problems. In the middle of the night, her heart briefly stopped beating. No one from the family was staying with her that first night. Mom told me about it when I visited on Sunday. She said the nurses panicked. I could tell it scared her too. That is when everyone realized the issue was not with her lungs, but her heart.

My mom's doctor called a family meeting on Sunday afternoon. Everyone was there except my sister who lives in Florida. The diagnosis was threefold: mitral valve prolapse, electrical impulses off, and aorta had calcification. Someone explained it to us in simpler terms: the valve was leaking (a door not shutting completely and letting blood flow back into chamber), the heart's rhythm was off, and there was not enough blood going in due to blockage. In essence, she would need a double pacemaker to keep her heart going.

In many ways, the doctor's communication was exemplary. Amati and Hannawa (2015) say "The key for successful end-of-life interactions is a careful, sensitive, and inclusive communication" (p. 242). The doctor emphasized the seriousness of her heart issues. He wanted the family to be clear about my mom's advanced directives. He explained that she was coded as "Do Not Resuscitate" (DNR). He described the techniques used when the emergency team performs resuscitation. He explained that her ribs might be broken in the process. He told us the results would not prolong her life much, but the procedure could seriously injure her. He told us that sometimes families, in their moment of stress and panic, ask the doctor to go against the patient's wishes. They ask him to take any possible actions. He said that in those moments he always has mixed feelings. He tries to honor the family's requests. He clearly needed us to understand Mom's wishes now, before crisis strikes. He wanted us to be a united front, difficult as that might be in the moment. Golden (2010) documents the dialectical issues of both certainty and control in the difficult negotiation of knowing the patient's wishes, yet questioning the role of family supporter.

Mom was reassuring. Again, her dual roles of both patient and practitioner were at the forefront of her decisions. She knew so much about the medical world. She knew what she did and did not want. The result of that meeting was that we understood Mom's wishes too. All except for my sister. It took us months recounting the events of those few weeks, to piece together how much my sister had missed; how that missing information affected her perceptions of the events as they unfolded.

The family stayed with Mom that day and discussed the diagnosis and potential options. We did not discuss the DNR directive specifically. Unspoken, it loomed large. Mom was not afraid of having a pacemaker installed. She told me the doctor might think she was afraid, but she was not. The surgery would need to occur at a larger hospital. She had already figured out how my dad could visit her there. He could park in the same garage they used for the wound care visits. She was so concerned about him, but not at all about herself. She was ready to move forward with whatever she needed to do to keep living.

I had to go back home on Monday. The semester was almost over, but I still had exams to give. When I visited Mom on my way out of town, I taught her how to take pictures on her cell phone. She practiced by taking shots of the spacious "hospice room." When I look at those photos now, it is hard to remember those moments before we knew what would eventually transpire in that room.

Mom went home on Monday with orders for oxygen, another upheaval to daily life. The long tubing allowed her to move throughout the house. By Tuesday, things were settling a bit. I was back home living my normal life, submitting final student grades and wrapping up the semester. The next day she experienced severe shortness of breath. Dad called 911. An ambulance took her back to the hospital. I left right away and arrived at the hospital around 11:00 pm. I stayed that night and from then on, someone in the family was with her night and day. There was talk of pneumonia spotted on a chest Xray. No one seemed certain of what was causing the breathing trouble.

During the night, her heart stopped again. Hospital staff flew into the room. I could feel the panic in the air. Someone ran to call her doctor. I was disoriented and confused. My mom was awake, but also seemed disoriented. A nurse tried to reassure me, telling me they would move Mom into the Intensive Care Unit (ICU) right away. Then, someone came back in the room and the flurry of activity instantly calmed. Looking back, I know that the call to the doctor prompted the drastic change in activity. There would be no rushing to the ICU. There would be no extreme treatments. This patient was DNR. Golden (2010) grappled with moments of uncertainty with regard to her dying grandmother's wishes and what that meant in the context of the hospital experiences.

No one explained anything to me. It would have been very helpful in the coming days if they had. I will never know if they could not tell me or just did not think about it. Amati and Hannawa (2014) include a need for ongoing communication as necessary element of end-of-life physician communication. I would agree. Maybe the hospital staff did not want to speak of the advanced directives in front of my mom. They did not know her the way I do. They did not know of her patient/practitioner duality. She might have been able to explain things to me, from her practitioner perspective. In the moment, my focus was on her as patient. She looked scared and frail. I held her hand for the rest of the night. I stroked it gently, trying to sooth the unsoothable.

The next morning Mom said she felt like she was "put in a bag and beaten with a ball bat." Later, she seemed to feel a bit better. She was talking and eating. My sister spent that next night with her. I needed to get back for one last exam on Friday, but I hated to leave her. My plan was to drive home, give the exam, and come right back. Some good-byes are harder than others. The memory of being there when her heart stopped kept me fully aware of the gravity of her situation. It felt like each moment was precious. As I headed out of town on country roads, I called my sister in Florida. My tears flowed freely. I told her she should come home.

My sister arrived from Florida on Saturday. That evening all three of her daughters sat with my mom watching one of her favorite TV shows. For a fleeting moment, things almost felt normal. Sunday was Mothers' Day. The irony was not lost on any of us. Many people came to visit that day. There were gifts, cards, and flowers. I brought Mom a book on local history. As we paged through the pictures, she shared more stories and I dutifully listened hard and took good notes in the margins. My husband and daughter drove over for the weekend. The mood was far from celebratory, but my mother's positivity brought a lightness to the room.

Mom was on morphine and occasionally it played with her sense of reality. I tried to comfort her when she was anxious and be her reality check. That night her heart stopped again. The episode took a lot out of her. As I sat holding her hand, she said, "I know why we had you. Because you are a good hand holder." Grassau and her colleagues examine "the flow of energy that moves between mothers and daughters as they navigate the meaning, significance and context of their connection as a mother is at the end of her life" (Grassau, 2014, p. 2; Grassau, Daly, Feldman, Shishis, and Tucker, 2016, p. 88). There were many moments in the coming days when I would feel that energy between us connecting and sustaining us.

My mom kept things light, but we both knew all that churned underneath the metaphor of handholding. My mom and I had been a great team for years.

I was her worker bee, tackling projects, doing chores, organizing, documenting, and helping her keep the household running and the family gatherings happening. Over the past few days, she and I talked about her concerns for my dad. He never handled the checkbook or the taxes. She was worried about how he would go on without her. There were moments when she knew what was coming much better than I did. I think she was trying to help me make sense, but it was too big for me to comprehend. I assured her that I would help my dad with anything he needed. I told her that she and I had been a fantastic team and that he and I could be a great team too.

It became clear that Mom's kidneys were beginning to fail. A portable heart monitor, about the size of large pocket calculator, had been tracking her heart rate and oxygen levels since she was admitted. Like any good nurse, she followed the levels closely. I think it gave her some illusion of control and tapped into her practitioner mindset. Unfortunately, her heart continued to stop for short moments of time. This, in turn, repeatedly frightened the nursing staff. We were puzzled when a nurse removed the monitor. The doctor had given me his cell phone number so, after much sisterly deliberation, I called to ask about the missing monitor. He returned my call quickly. I do not recall the details of the conversation. He reassured me that someone would reconnect the monitor. At the time, we assumed this must have been a mistake. In retrospect, I think he knew the end was near, but would not (or could not) find the way to share this information.

This was another moment where direct communication could have helped us make sense of our situation. None of us wanted our mother to die. However, our lack of information about her current situation had no power to prevent that from happening. When Kellett (2017) describes his uncertainty when experiencing vision loss, he states, "some sort of vision loss coach would have been useful in helping me understand things, and keeping things in perspective" (p. 30). There were so many times during the last days of my mother's life that I felt a similar need and an accompanying frustration.

I stayed with Mom that night. In the early morning hours, the night nurse gave me a hug at the end of her shift. It was both comforting and heavy with the gravity of our situation. Later when I woke, Mom was unresponsive. I called my sisters. Later, Mom's minister entered the hospital room and she suddenly woke up. He prayed and talked with her for a while. After he left she ordered breakfast and as we talked she cheerfully said, "I can't wait to see them!" Confused, but assuming she meant family who would be visiting soon, I asked "Who?" She replied "Mother and Daddy." I was stunned and uncertain how to respond. Both had been gone for many years. In that moment, I knew enough about end-of-life experiences to appreciate the significance of what had occurred. I now know so much more about the complexities of final conversations (Keeley, 2016; Keely & Yingling, 2007) and communication at the end-of-life (Nussbaum, Giles, & Worthington, 2015).

Later, with family gathered by her side, she smiled and talked with a brightness in her eyes that had not been there before. The conversations were heart-felt and poignant. She exchanged "I love yous" with my dad, a rare public display of affection in our family. There was an ethereal look in her eyes. I assumed this was some sort of "final conversation" and the end was near. I had no idea what to expect as we moved forward. Again, I yearned for a coach, an advisor, or someone to tell me what was coming next.

Mom slept most of the day, waking in the afternoon. She asked for lemon ice and I sat by her side, scraping the frozen contents and feeding her like a baby. Neither of us minded. The cold treat was soothing to her and the intimacy comforted me. That afternoon, they wheeled her bed to the hospice room we had occupied only a week earlier. I kissed her forehead as they rolled her away. She replied with a smile and a childlike "Thank you!"

The last few days in that hospice room were both beautiful and horrifying. Mom lost consciousness sometime Monday night. My sisters, brother, and I kept vigil day and night. Dad came for visits, but slept at home. We played hymns for her through the night. We tried singing and reciting Psalm 23. It was her favorite. However, Sunday school had been too long ago and we failed miserably. I am sure she agreed that it was the thought that counts. We rubbed lotion on her arms and legs. We caressed her cheek and smoothed her hair. Most importantly, we made sure someone was always holding both of her hands. My family's displays of affection are limited. Nevertheless, I felt a need to touch her. I found myself saying, "I am going to give you a kiss on the forehead because I can" to account for my behavior.

The nursing staff cared for Mom with such compassion. They came in routinely to shift her positioning, support her with pillows and swaddle her in blankets. Even as her body was failing, we all gathered to support her and love her into the next realm. We joked that she was like the energizer bunny because her heart continued to beat steadily. Keeley and Baldwin (2013) see the act of giving permission as a key part of positive communication during end of life conversations. Over the course of those days, we told her she could let go whenever she was ready. We assured her we would be okay. A little after 2:00 pm on Wednesday, I was holding her hand and rubbing her shoulder. I patted her chest and said, "It's okay to let go, energizer bunny." I saw her eyes opening and called to my dad, seated on the other side of the bed. Everyone leapt up and stared into her eyes, open for the first time in a day and a half. The doctor later said it must have taken all the strength she had left to open her eyes. I remember saying "there are those beautiful blue eyes" and she shifted her gaze in my direction for the briefest of moments. Then, she was gone.

My mom's life may have ended that day, but her story lives on. It is the story of our mother-daughter relationship, the story of the power of positivity, the story of navigating the dialectic pulls of being both patient and practitioner, in times of change/decline and stability, when loss of autonomy leads to new levels of connectedness, when what was once private becomes public, and when resilience balances fragility.

REFERENCES

Amati, R., & Hannawa, A. F. (2014). Relational Dialectics Theory: Disentangling physician-perceived tensions of end-of-life communication. *Health Communication*, *29*(10), 962–73. doi: 10.1080/10410236.2013.815533.

Amati, R., & Hannawa, A. F. (2015). Physician-perceived contradictions in end-of-life communication: Toward a self-report measurement scale. *Health Communication*, *30*(3), 241–50. doi: 10.1080/10410236.2013.841532.

Baxter, L. A. & Montgomery B. M. (1996) *Relating: Dialogues and dialectics.* New York: Guilford.

Birch, C. L. & Heckler, M. A. (1996). *Who says?: Essays on pivotal issues in contemporary storytelling.* Little Rock, AR: August House.

Cardow, A. (2017). Returning to work a better nurse. *Canadian Nurse*, *113*(5), 44.

Celaya, E. (2018). When nurses need to be nursed. *British Journal of Nursing*, *27*(9), 500.

Edward, K., Giandinoto, J. & McFarland, J. (2017). Analysis of the experiences of nurses who return to nursing after cancer. *British Journal of Nursing*, *26*(21), 1170–175.

Ehrenreich (2001, November). Welcome to cancerland. *Harper's Magazine*, 303(1818), pp. 43–53.

Fisher, C. L. (2011). "Her pain was my pain" Mothers and daughters sharing the breast cancer journey. In M. Miller-Day (Ed.) *Family communication, connections, and health transitions: Going through this together.* (pp 57–76) New York: Peter Lang.

Fisher, C. L., Miller-Day, M., Nussbaum, J. F. (2013). Healing through healthy doses of positivity: Mothers' and daughters' positive communication when coping with breast cancer. In M. J. Pitts & T. J. Socha (Eds.) *Positive communication in health and wellness.* (pp. 98–113), New York: Peter Lang.

Golden, M. A. (2010). Dialectical contradictions experienced when a loved one is dying in a hospital setting. *Omega: Journal of Death & Dying*, *62*(1), 31–49. doi: 10.2190/OM.62.1.b.

Gottschall, J. (2012). *The storytelling animal: How stories make us human.* Boston: Houghton Mifflin Harcourt.

Grassau, P. A. (2014). *Navigating the cathexis: Mothers and daughters and end of life* (Unpublished doctoral dissertation). University of Toronto, Toronto.

Grassau, P., Daly, S., Feldman, J., ShiShis, L., & Tucker, T. (2016). P096 Navigating the cathexis: Mothers and daughters in end of life and bereavement. *Journal of Pain and Symptom Management*, *52*(6), e88–e89. doi:10.1016/j.jpainsymman.2016.10.182.

Keeley, M. P. (2016). Family communication at the end of life. *Journal of Family Communication*, *16*(3), 189–97.

Keeley M. P. and Baldwin, P. (2013). Final conversations: Positive communication at the end of life. In M. J. Pitts & T. J. Socha (Eds.) *Positive communication in health and wellness.* (pp. 190–203), New York: Peter Lang.

Keeley, M. P. & Generous, M. A. (2015). The challenges of final conversations: Dialectical tensions during end-of-life family communication. *Southern Communication Journal*, *80*(5), 377–87.

Keeley, M. P. & Yingling, J. M. 2007). *Final conversations: Helping the living and the dying talk to each other.* Acton, MA: VanderWyk & Burnham.

Kellett, P. M. (2017). *Patienthood and communication: A personal narrative of eye disease and vision loss.* New York: Peter Lang.

Knight, A. (2018). From nurse to service user: a personal cancer narrative. *British Journal of Nursing*, *27*(4), s18–s21.

Miller, V. D., & Knapp, M. L. (1986). Communication paradoxes and the maintenance of living relationships with the dying. *Journal of Family Issues, 7*(3), 255–75. doi:10.1177/019251386007003003

Montgomery, B. M. & Baxter, L. A. (Eds.) (1998) *Dialectical approaches to studying personal relationships*. Mahwah, NJ: Lawrence Erlbaum Associates.

Nussbaum, J. F., Giles, H., & Worthington, A. K. (2015). *Communication at the end of life*. New York: Peter Lang.

O'Hara, L. L. S. (2017). Discursive struggles in "diabetes management": A case study using Baxter's Relational Dialectics 2.0. *Western Journal of Communication, 81*(3), 320–40. doi:10.1080/10570314.2016.1241425.

Pitts, M. J. & Socha, T. J. (2013) *Positive communication in health and wellness*. New York: Peter Lang.

Scholl, J. C. (2013). Humor as a tool, not the therapy: A preliminary model of humor in health communication. In M. J. Pitts & T. J. Socha (Eds.) *Positive communication in health and wellness*. (pp. 43–62), New York: Peter Lang.

Socha, T. J. & Pitts, M. J. (2012). *The positive side of interpersonal communication*. New York: Peter Lang.

Sullivan, C. F. (2013). Positive relational communication: Impact on health. In M. J. Pitts & T. J. Socha (Eds.) *Positive communication in health and wellness*. (pp. 29–42), New York: Peter Lang.

Chapter Twelve

A Narrative Account of Father-Daughter Conversations Near the End of His Life

Deanna F. Womack

As we waited in the physician's office, I asked my father to sign the Veterans Administration form designating me to manage his finances. I had been very pleased when I received the letter from the Veterans Administration awarding my father, a World War II veteran, current and accumulated benefits to help cover his assisted living costs. However, there was no check with the letter because my father's physician had declared him mentally incompetent to manage his financial affairs. So, the letter came with a form requiring him to sign designating someone else to manage his finances. As he always had, my father read the form before he signed it. When he came to the section about mental incompetence, he asked, "Is that me?" I responded, "Yes." "Oh," he said with a facial expression of surprise, and quietly signed the form.

Although brief, this was a difficult conversation because my father had earned an MBA and was a CPA and CMA (Certified Management Accountant). As I waited for him to sign, I remembered the many trips he had made to New York when I was a teenager to sell bonds on behalf of the city and county governments for which he worked. In one new job, my father arranged an automatic transfer of funds every Friday night out of the government checking accounts into savings because the monies would not be needed over the weekend. Early every Monday morning the funds went back to the checking accounts. By moving unused funds into the savings accounts every weekend, he had earned millions of dollars in interest for the government. But now, to receive the VA stipend he had been awarded, he had to agree that he could no longer manage his own finances.

This conversation was emblematic of the kinds of discussions my father and I engaged in as he neared the end of his life. Although he resided in an assisted living facility, I had to provide transportation for physicians' visits and treatment. My brother lived in California, and we had no family near us in Atlanta. In fact, we had very few family members at all because both my father and mother were only children. So, my father and I were alone on these trips to the doctor, and that gave us many chances to talk privately.

This chapter is a personal narrative evoking themes of the conversations my father and I had about four topic areas: changes in the way people treated him as he grew older, constructing a new identity after short-term memory loss left him with diminished capacity, negotiating patienthood with him as he required more and more medical care, and the role reversal that occurs between aging parents and their adult children who become central caregivers.

Much of the literature about communicating with older adults focuses on interactions between older adults and those of other generations. Communication accommodation theory (CAT) (Giles, Coupland, & Coupland, 1991; Giles, 2008) forms the basis for most of these articles from the communication discipline. CAT describes the ways that conversational partners adjust their communication behaviors to each other. The theory also explains why speakers adjust in particular ways to their partners' verbal and nonverbal patterns. Throughout the conversation, speakers evaluate their partners' motives and the conversation pattern and consciously or non-consciously adjust their responses in one of four ways based on the speakers' motives and attributions of their partners' motives (Giles, 2008). First, speakers who converge express desires to gain social approval by mimicking their partners' verbal and nonverbal patterns, such as adjusting their language by repeating partners' jargon. Convergence is designed to minimize social distance between partners to express the desire to affiliate, even though partners may not be consciously aware of this goal (Muir, Joinson, Cotterill, & Dewdney, 2016). Empirical research has shown that those whose partners accommodate them tend to judge them positively. For example, they like the partners more and are more likely to judge them as similar to themselves (Giles, Taylor, & Bourhis, 1973). In contrast, partners who diverge, "inappropriately [adjust their behavior] for participants in an interaction" (Gasiorek & Giles, 2012, p. 312), for example, by emphasizing differences between their communicative behaviors and their partners'. Partners are likely to consider conversational partners who diverge to be impolite or even hostile (Gasiorek & Giles, 2012).

As with divergence, there are other forms of conversation that are likely to be viewed less favorably than convergence. Non-accommodation, or failure to converge, may be interpreted negatively by recipients "as suggesting that they are not worthy of the sender's respect or positive regard," especially between members of different language groups or dialects (Giles, 2008, p. 124).

Research indicates two forms, under-accommodation and over-accommodation, are especially likely to affect intergenerational conversations. Under-accommodation is perceived as insufficient adjustment to a partner's conversational style. As discussed and cited in Giles (2008):

> Many complex factors can lead to mis-carrying out accommodative dispositions, despite positive intentions. For example, many American young people claim difficulties with intergenerational relations. . . . Part of the problem is that older people are seen as under-accommodative. Not only do they seem to express negative stereotypes about today's youth, but they do not sufficiently attend to, and neither are they willing apparently to appreciate, the needs and messages of their younger counterparts (Giles & Williams, 1994). At the same time, elders are heard to be overly verbose about the "good old days" yet also talk excessively about painful past events such as illnesses and bereavements (Barker, 2007). Studies show that such disclosures are very difficult for recipients to manage . . . and are attributed by younger people to decrements in cognitive and communicative functioning (Coupland, Coupland, & Giles, 1991).
>
> However, when analyzing actual intergenerational discourse, more palatable social explanations are discovered. A potent one is self-handicapping, in the sense that older people are making a statement about the vibrancy of their present physical and subjective well-being, even though they have endured debilitating events. The message intended is more one of heroic coping and healthy adjustment than any morose obsession with past problems. Typically, though, it is rarely interpreted this way by younger people; older folks are often oblivious to the destructive under-accommodating premise that such painful divulgences can instill in those more youthful. (pp. 122–23)

Over-accommodation (Williams & Nussbaum, 2001) is another feature often found in intergenerational conversations. Older people may feel that younger people patronize them by talking to them as children by speaking very slowly, using simplistic grammar, exaggerated enunciations, and overly emphatic nonverbal behavior such as too-frequent smiles, head nods, or touches (Ryan, Hummert, & Boich, 1995; Nussbaum, Hummert, Williams, & Harwood, 1996; Nussbaum, Pitts, Huber, Raup Krieger, & Ohs, 2005). Over-accommodation may negatively affect older adults (Giles, 2008):

> Feeling condescended to and controlled by many different younger people across many different social contexts can be sapping of people's self-esteem and also accelerate physical demise. That said, this practice is often borne out of nurturing, benevolent, intent and has been shown to be appreciated by the very old and frail. (p. 123)

It is clear from the CAT research that both under-accommodation and over-accommodation are likely to be misunderstood in the context of intergenerational interpersonal conversations.

A second theory that can be applied to conversations between those of different age cohorts is the communication theory of identity (Hecht, 1993). As cited in Hecht (1993) reflecting anthropological, sociological, and psychological perspectives, the communication theory of identity is grounded in the premise that:

> identity is inherently a communicative process and must be understood as a transaction in which messages are exchanged (Collier & Thomas, 1988; Shotter & Gergen, 1989). These messages are symbolic linkages between and among people that, at least in part, are enactments of identity. Even when identity is largely symbolic (Gans, 1979), communication rituals are used to create and express it. (p. 78)

The communication theory of identity is based on eight basic assumptions, one of which is that identities are both enduring and changing. As older adults retire and perhaps move to assisted living or other communal residences and make new friends, it is reasonable to expect that identities may change at least somewhat with these major life changes since identities "are codes that are expressed in conversations and define membership in communities." They also "prescribe modes of appropriate and effective communication" (Hecht, 1993, p. 79). Identities may be understood through four frames of reference that are "means of interpreting reality that provide a perspective for understanding the social world (Hecht, 1984)" (from Hecht, 1993, p. 81).

The four frames are the personal, enacted, relational, and communal frames. Viewed through the personal frame, identity is a "characteristic of the individual stored as self-cognitions, feelings about self, and/or a spiritual sense of self being." Identities "are meanings ascribed to the self by others in the social world" (Hecht, 1993, p. 79). Enacted identities are performed through communication and may be identified by messages individuals send. It is important to note that in the enactment frame, identities emerge through this communication performance. Through the relationship frame, identities are social and enacted in relationships. There are four levels of relational identity. The first level, ascribed relational identity, consists of the identities we develop by internalizing how others see us (Jung & Hecht, 2004). The second emerges in relationships with other people. Because people have multiple identities, identities at the third level exist in relationship to one's other identities. At the fourth level of relationship identities, "relationship itself can be a unit of identity," for example, the relationships of father and daughter (Jung & Hecht, 2004, p. 266). Communal identities, the final frame, emerge from networks or groups with which one is associated. For my father, one salient communal identity was that of a member of the Masonic Lodge.

Identities become dynamic because of the interpenetration of frames. Frames can be consistent or inconsistent with each other. They may even sometimes be contradictory. Discrepant frames result in "identity gaps" that are unavoidable in communication (Jung & Hecht, 2004). Jung and Hecht (2004) investigate two important identity gaps. The gap between the personal and ascribed identities refers to discrepancies in the way people view themselves and the way others view them. The gap between personal and enacted identities refers to a discrepancy between a person's felt identity and the way a person presents him or herself to others. In their study, Jung and Hecht (2004) explore the relationship gaps between personal and ascribed identities and between personal and enacted identities. They confirmed that these two identity gaps were negatively associated with three important communication outcomes: feeling understood, communication satisfaction, and conversational appropriateness and effectiveness.

Thus, both these theories describe and explain concepts and events that may affect older adults. As Hummert (2009) details, communication research distinguishes ineffective from effective communication behaviors and connects them with desirable communication outcomes. Thus, nursing home workers and family members may be taught that patronizing talk (overaccommodation) directed toward older adults is harmful to their self-esteem and thus may negatively affect their personal and ascribed relational identities or widen identity gaps that physical changes brought about by the aging process may already have created. Throughout this personal narrative, communication accommodation theory and the communication theory of identity will be used to highlight features of conversations with my father that reflect communication outcomes.

NAVIGATING CHANGES

My father was a proud man who was used to being in charge. Someone meeting my father for the first time would not likely detect the evidence of diminished capacity, other than his obvious loss of hearing. The only evidence of incompetence was that he had lost much of his short-term memory after a stroke. For example, after he moved from one apartment in assisted living to another, he was having delivery problems with the daily newspaper. I stopped by to check and asked my father if he had received the paper that morning. "No," he said. As I was leaving, I noticed the current newspaper on the floor by his favorite chair where he had dropped it. His diminished capacity was apparent only to someone who had known him before the stroke or someone, like his primary care physician, who saw him more frequently as his health declined. My father had fought in Italy in World War II, and the physician had a surname of Italian origin. Every time Dad visited his doctor he noticed her name badge and asked if she was Italian. She replied that the name was her husband's name. His parents were Italian. The same conversation occurred during each visit. That doctor patiently answered my father's questions every time. Because my father often did not notice instances of his short-term memory loss, he was unaware of the gap between his personal identity of competence and the enacted identity of forgetfulness that others ascribed to him (Jung & Hecht, 2004). While this gap could have caused him distress, the short-term memory loss apparently prevented him from recalling instances in which he did not act competently in the judgments of others.

At the end of our visits, I often took my father out to lunch as a treat. Eventually, my father needed to use a wheelchair when he left the assisted living facility. That was when I understood what he meant when he told me, "When you get old you become invisible." When he used a walker, servers asked him for his order. But when he eventually needed to use a wheelchair, the server usually talked only to me as though he were not sitting at the table. They asked me for his order as well as mine and gave me the check. While I never heard an example of baby talk or other over-accommodation addressed to my father, Giles (2008) also mentions over-accommodation in the context of persons with disabilities. "Addressing the companion of someone about the latter's needs and not the physically challenged person is a problematic feature of inter-ability encounters" (pp. 123–24). Because we never had a conversation other than the comment reported above about my father's reaction to servers addressing me instead of him, I do not know whether or how much the emotions associated with his personal identity or a conflict between his identity before and after using the wheelchair affected his self-esteem or caused other communication problems. He was certainly aware of becoming invisible.

By the time my father was using a wheelchair, he was willing to let me pay the check with his credit card. We had had several lunches in which he could not remember whether the server had come with a check and he had paid it or whether we were still waiting for the check. So, he let me take over paying because I could keep track of the process and make sure we did pay, but only once. We switched from paying with cash to using his credit card for the same reason: it was easier to keep track of the process. The communication theory of identity (Hecht, 1993) suggests that my father's personal identity likely changed as he became aware that he couldn't remember events well enough to be in charge of paying. Thus, his identity likely shifted toward his perceiving himself less competent in money matters, at which he had once excelled. Though he had never been diagnosed with dementia, he was aware that he had some cognitive impairment. He told me, "I don't think as clearly as I used to." I believe this realization made it easier for him to let me pay his bills even though he had much more financial knowledge than I did. Around this time, I bought him a beginner's Sudoku book thinking he might like the game and it might strengthen his cognitive abilities. He looked at the book and declined it. I believe he decided it would be too difficult for him and therefore more frustrating than fun because, after I had explained the rules, he said, "I can't do that." This conversation indicated he was aware of new limitations on his cognitive abilities and illustrates the dynamic nature of identities (Hecht, 1993).

RECONSTRUCTING A NEW IDENTITY

Aware that he was not able to think as well as he had before the stroke, my father needed to construct a new sense of identity. If his identity had not changed, his dominant personality would have made it very difficult for me to help with his finances and make decisions related to his healthcare. Narrative is an appropriate way to investigate identity for several reasons. First, Ladegaard (2012) notes that narratives perform the psychological function of helping narrators make sense of their situations. Second, narratives and identities are embedded in a temporal and cultural context (Ladegaard, 2012). Therefore, identities are, "continuously remade, highly situational, sometimes contradictory" (Ladegaard, 2012, p. 451). According to Benwell and Stokoe (2006), "The practice of narration involves the 'doing' of identity, and because we can tell different stories we can construct different versions of self" (p. 138). Just as my father's earlier identity had emphasized competence and integrity in managing government finances, his new identity emphasized giving up control in many ways and recognizing that he needed help in making decisions.

His new identity often contradicted elements of the identity he had established before the stroke, creating an identity gap (Jung & Hecht, 2004) between old and new personal identities. While I do not remember him ever asking me what he should do, he did often rely on me to negotiate treatment options with the physicians and implement their suggestions. During the last six months of his life, my father developed a skin rash that the dermatologist was unable to treat successfully with creams or pills. The last choice of treatment was a therapy that required him to stand completely naked in a circular light booth for ten minutes or more. My father did not comment or ask questions while the physician and I discussed that the treatment depended on me to transport him to the appropriate medical office twice a week. The light booth was in a very small treatment room with a bench for me to sit on just outside of the booth. My father undressed in a separate closet area and approached the booth wearing only his undershorts. Once inside the light booth, he had to drop his shorts. The treatment itself went smoothly, but he had difficulty bending down far enough to reach his shorts to get dressed. On the first visits we had a nurse or medical assistant to help us, but I realized we needed to find a way to help him dress on his own. So, I rigged up two binder clips, each attached to a three foot long piece of ribbon. He attached the clips to his shorts and wrapped the loops at the top ends of the ribbon around his hands. He dropped the shorts, then, after the treatment, used the ribbons around his wrists to pull the shorts up so that he could put them on by himself. We used this method for the next two months during treatment. My rigged-up system for helping my father raise his shorts preserved his modesty by enabling him to dress and undress independently. He was pleased with the arrangement, and it made us both more comfortable with the procedure. I believe this was because it narrowed the gap between his prideful personal identity and the enacted identity of someone who needed his daughter's help to get dressed.

NEGOTIATING PATIENTHOOD NEEDS

My father and I never had an extended conversation about his new identity. I was able to use fragments of conversations and phrases to construct an idea of how his identity had changed at the end of life. My father had a very dominant personality that softened as he began to depend on me and to trust my judgment about major healthcare and financial decisions. Before he moved into assisted living, people who knew him or even just interacted once or twice with him perceived him as someone very capable of managing government finances. After he began to use a wheelchair on outings, he became invisible to those we encountered. Because he told me he felt invisible as he became older and that he was not able to think as clearly as he had before his stroke, I infer that his identity changed from someone who was highly competent to someone who was less competent. His interactions with others changed from those of an agent, someone who acts, to those of a patient, someone who is acted upon. Without argument or discussion, he signed a form saying that he was mentally incompetent to manage his financial affairs, giving me the power to manage them for him. He changed from someone who could help others to someone who regularly required help. As a teenager, I remember him always taking charge and making decisions for others in the family. After the stroke, he willingly let me take control and did what I told him to do without questioning my choices. By the time he had been diagnosed with prostate cancer, he was aware that he was sometimes not thinking clearly, could not remember recent events (though he clearly remembered events from World War II), and had begun to think of himself as a person who needed help and guidance from others. He realized he could no longer be independent. His identity changed to someone who needed to depend on others, another example of the dynamic nature of personal identity (Jung & Hecht, 2004) throughout the lifespan.

MANAGING ROLE REVERSAL

As the eldest child, the only daughter, and the only relative living in the same city, I experienced role reversal as my parents aged. As U.S. life expectancies have increased (CDC, 2018), many older adults experience a slow decline in abilities to manage their own affairs. Typically, these responsibilities shift to children or other relatives, so that the child takes care of the parent. This change in roles can create identity gaps between enacted and personal identities and between personal and relational identities (Jung & Hecht, 2004). In role reversal, the personal identity shifts from "the one in charge of helping" to "the one needing help." Negotiating this role reversal with my father after he suffered a stroke and entered an assisted living residence was both challenging and interesting.

After my father had lived in the residence for about two years, he had a car accident that greatly increased his auto insurance costs. He was eighty-three, and he no longer had the excellent sense of direction he had had when he was younger. I was afraid he would get lost and not be able to find his way back or know how to contact me, so we discussed whether he should continue to drive. My father was not fully aware of the impact of his memory loss at this point. He had not yet accepted the effect his weakening vision and hearing, and his diminished sense of direction, had had on his driving skills. We discussed the increased insurance costs because of the accident. Hearing the cost convinced him that he should stop driving. My father believed there had been a traffic ticket associated with the accident, which he thought he had paid. I pointed out that if he could not find the ticket and was not sure that he had paid it that was an indication his memory loss might affect his driving as well. He also frequently lost his car keys and locked himself out of his car or apartment, events that had occurred throughout his lifetime. Therefore, after we agreed that he probably should not drive, I just took the keys. My father assumed he had lost the keys and searched for them several times. Eventually, he gave up looking and became resigned to depending on me for transportation.

With my children in elementary school, my father and I also discussed how to balance my care for him while I was also caring for my daughters and working full time. I tried to stop by the assisted living residence about twice a week to visit with him there. I also took him out for lunch as often as I could. Even though the facility planned many activities, my father wanted to get out more often, especially after he stopped driving and depended on me for transportation. I told him that I was doing the best I could, and I explained the activities that my children were involved in. His response was, "They come first," and I agreed that they had to because they were so little. The fact that he had told me they should be my first priority allowed me to feel less guilty.

This conversation was representative of the kinds of communication my father and I had as he approached the end of his life and I became his caretaker. He did not question individual decisions or discuss details so much as he emphasized principles I should follow. Once when we were discussing using his bank account to reimburse me for expenses, rather than telling me how much to withdraw or asking questions about various amounts, he simply said, "You'll do what's right." As an accountant and auditor, honesty had been one of his hallmark values both professionally and personally. This conversation indicated to me that he trusted me and that he thought my definition of "what's right" would be like his. So, he emphasized the value involved and trusted me to interpret and implement it.

The most frequent but one of the briefest exchanges we had on every trip involved my father thanking me for taking him to the doctor, out to lunch, or wherever we had been. Sometimes he thanked me several times on one trip. He told me he realized that sometimes he repeated his thanks, but he wanted to be sure he remembered to thank me. My father, an only child, had taken care of his mother, who had asthma and other health problems. Unlike him, she never expressed gratitude. Instead she berated him and told all her friends that my father neglected her because he could not do as much as she wanted. So, I believe his own experience of caregiving informed the way he behaved when the roles were reversed. He was always careful to thank me for my help.

When he thanked me, I always responded the same way: "I'm glad to be able to do it, Daddy." In these conversations, my ability "to do it" had two levels of meaning for me. First, for example, I was glad that I had a flexible work schedule that allowed me to take him for light box treatments twice every week. And second, I was grateful that my parents had moved from North Carolina to Atlanta to live with us before they had to move to assisted living. It was much easier for me to meet their needs when they lived a mile away than it would have been to go back and forth to North Carolina when they needed something, even though they had a group of friends in North Carolina who would have been willing to help.

As I reflect on it, my father's psychological and identity transition from someone in charge to someone who depended on others, was gradual and relatively smooth. Unlike friends whose parents became paranoid and refused to discuss finances or let them help pay bills, I never had to fight with my father about decisions. He trusted me and willingly delegated his choices about money and healthcare to me. The smooth shifts in his identity helped me to help him, and he seemed to accept the more passive role of care receiver. We were able to adjust to his healthcare challenges as well as to the role reversal demanded of both of us. Although we had frequently fought each other when I was a teenager, thankfully we cooperated well to manage the changes that his growing older required.

REFERENCES

Barker, D. J. P. (2007). The origins of the developmental origins theory. *Journal of internal medicine*, *261*(5), 412–417.
Benwell, B., & Stokoe, E. (2006). *Identity and discourse*. Edinburgh, UK: University of Edinburgh Press.
Collier, M. J., & Thomas, M. (1988). Cultural identity: An interpretive perspective, pp. 99–120 in Kim, Young Yun, & Gudykunst, William B. (Eds.), *Theories in Intercultural Communication*. Sage.
Cortazzi, M. (2001). Narrative analysis in ethnography. In P. Atkinson, A. Coffey, S. Delamont, J. Lofland, & E. Lofland (Eds). *Handbook of ethnography* (pp. 384–94). Thousand Oaks, CA: Sage.
Coupland, J., Coupland, N., & Giles, H. (1991) (Eds.). Sociolinguistic issues in ageing. *Ageing and Society*, *11*(2), 99–243.
Centers for Disease Control. (2018, Sept. 18. Retrieved from https://www.cdc.gov/nchs/.
Gans, H. J. (1979). Symbolic ethnicity: The future of ethnic groups and cultures in America. *Ethnic and Racial Studies*, *2*: 1–20.
Gasiorek, J., & Giles, H. (2012). Effects of inferred motive on evaluations of nonaccommodative communication. *Human Communication Research*, *38*, 309–31.
Giles, H. (2008). Accommodating translational research. *Journal of Applied Communication Research*, *36*, 121–27.
Giles, H., Coupland, N., & Coupland, J. (1991). Accommodation theory: Communication, context, and consequence. In H. Giles, J. Coupland, & N. Coupland (Eds.), *Contexts of accommodation: Developments in applied linguistics* (pp. 1–68). Cambridge: Cambridge University Press.
Giles, H., Taylor, D. M., & Bourhis, R. (1973). Towards a theory of interpersonal accommodation through language: Some Canadian data. *Language in Society*, *2*, 177–92.
Giles, H., & Williams, A. (1994) Patronizing the young: Forms and evaluations. *International Journal of Aging & Human Development*, *39*, 33–53.
Hecht, M. L. (1984). Satisfying communication and relationship labels: Intimacy and length of relationship as perceptual frames of naturalistic conversations. *Western Journal of Speech Communication*, *48*, 201–16.
Hecht, M. L. (1993). 2002: A research odyssey: Toward the development of a communication theory of identity. *Communication Monographs*, *60*, 76–82.
Hummert, M. L. (2009). Not just preaching to the choir: Communication scholarship does make a difference. *Journal of Applied Communication Research*, *37*, 215–24.
Jung, E., & Hecht, M. L. (2004). Elaborating the communication theory of identity: Identity gaps and communication outcomes. *Communication Quarterly*, *52*, 265–83.
Ladegaard, H. J. (2012). The discourse of powerlessness and repression: Identity construction in domestic helper narratives. *Journal of Sociolinguistics*, *16*, 450–82. doi.org/10.1111/j.1467-9841.2012.00541.x.
Muir, K., Joinson, A., Cotterill, R., & Dewdney, N. (2016). Characterizing the linguistic chameleon: Personal and social correlates of linguistic style accommodation. *Human Communication Research*, *42*, 462–85.
Nussbaum, J. F., Hummert, M. L., Williams, A., & Harwood, J. (1996). Communication and older adults. *Communication Yearbook*, *19*, 1–47.
Nussbaum, J. F., Pitts, M. J., Huber, F. N., Raup Krieger, & Ohs, J. E. (2005). Ageism and ageist language across the lifespan: Intimate relationships and non-intimate interactions. *Journal of Social Issues*, *61*, 287–306.

Ryan, E. B., Hummert, M. L., & Boich, L. H. (1995). Communication predicaments of aging: Patronizing behavior toward older adults. *Journal of Language and Social Psychology, 14*, 144–66.

Shotter, J., & Gergen, K. J. (1989) (Eds.). *Texts of identity*. London: Sage.

Williams, A., & Nussbaum, J. F. (2001). *Intergenerational communication across the lifespan*. Mahwah, NJ: Erlbaum.

Chapter Thirteen

A Narrative Legacy of Family Caregiving

Elizabeth A. Spencer

In early 2013, my brother and I sat in a neurologist's office with our sixty-two-year-old mother. The physician had just given her a verbal cognitive test about dates, basic mathematical ability, and simple memory exercises. She was flush with embarrassment and fury. She could not remember the president's name. She did not know what year it was. She stumbled over numbers as she tried to calculate 40 minus 7. It was too uncomfortable to watch. The tension was so thick I was nauseous.

He began talking about the medications he was prescribing. I interrupted and asked what the diagnosis was.

"Alzheimer's disease," the doctor said. It was as if he kicked me in the stomach. I felt as if all the air had left my lungs.

My mother gasped and stammered, "Well, what good did *that* do?!" she yelled as she stormed out into the hallway.

That day was a milestone, a turning point; a shift in her and our interwoven life course trajectories (Elder, 1998; Karp, 1997; Pound, Gompertz, & Ebrahim, 1998). Illness impacts individual, relational/social, and collective group identities. By seeing oneself as sick, this creates an illness identity in which it is difficult to separate self from illness (Karp, 1997). Entangled in this is a required acknowledgment that oneself is damaged. Illness diagnosis can be an identity marker, a turning point of a shift in identity from healthy to sick. A critical importance of an official diagnosis (i.e., labeling of an experience or state) is now the acceptance that you "have" something (Karp, 1997). Diagnosis can be both a frightening experience and a relief. It can create feelings of certainty and safety. Diagnosis can also be a significant biographical disruption (Bury, 1982).

That day in the neurologist's office was not the beginning of this journey. We had experienced years of mother's confusion, uncertainty, and concern. But that day, we finally had a diagnosis. We had an official label to put on what we saw and had experienced. My brother and I had been trying for years to get some help for our mother; trying to figure out what was wrong, trying to find some answers. We started seeing the hint of some unusual behavior and the decline of her functioning ability in 2005. She was fifty-five at that time.

She was always very independent. A single mother, she had to work hard to provide for us. The youngest of seven children, she was heartbroken seeing her parents and each of her siblings pass away. As she lost that extended support, my brother and I began to notice some concerning changes. By 2010, we could no longer deny something was wrong. She could not keep a job. She would not pay her bills. She was easily upset and had irrational emotional outbursts. One evening, in those early days, I took her to an ice cream shop. That night they did not have her favorite flavor. She yelled at the clerk and stomped out of the store.

In the early years of her illness, as our concern was growing, we tried repeatedly to get Mom to move to a maintenance free residence. By 2010, her house was in shambles. She could not take care of her home any longer. We asked her, pleaded with her, to sell her house and move to an apartment. But the more we asked, the angrier she got. "I will NEVER leave my home," she seethed through gritted teeth.

Aging in place is a foundational principle recognized and examined by gerontologists and aging and health researchers and practitioners (Greenfield, Oberlink, Scharlach, Neal, & Stafford, 2015; Satariano, Scharlach, & Lindeman, 2014). The conceptualization of place has an impact upon identity (Proshansky, Fabian, & Kaminoff, 1983; Vignoles, Schwartz, & Luyckx, 2011). Attachment to a personal residence can be viewed as a marker of identity. Home can represent a place of safety and refuge. It can be a physical location with material artifacts (Belk, 1988; Mittal, 2006) where one perceives of oneself as "healthy," as opposed to a healthcare facility, a place where one is "ill" (Karp, 1997). Physical environment, illness, and identity are intertwined (Karp, 1997).

The issue of identity's interwoven nature to place became one of the major elements of concern and contention in our family. My mother's home and the attachment she had to the land it was built on held a powerful connection. Throughout our childhood we heard stories of her father, our grandfather, farming the land and helping her build her home. She built it in small phases, piece by piece. She paid cash for each phase of construction, working as a waitress, never taking a mortgage. Her home was a symbol of pride and familial connection. In her eyes, it symbolized her family's legacy and represented her identity as an autonomous and self-reliant woman.

My mother, Georgia Ann Bradley, had fiery red curly hair and was as fiercely independent and determined as might stereotypically be expected of redheads. She was proud of her hair color that she had inherited from her father and beamed with pride when both of her grandsons were born with red locks. She was tenacious. We knew when she said she was not ready to leave her home, that this was a battle we would not win in 2010.

Illness can create a biographical disruption for families. A biographical disruption occurs when illness disrupts the normal rules of reciprocity and mutual support within families (Bury, 1982). As caregiving demands increase there is a breaching of traditional family role boundaries. Serious illnesses force reevaluation and redefinition of both individual and family identities (Charmaz, 1999). Illness can cause a rethinking down to the foundational level of a family member's personal identity and question the mobilization of collective family resources (Bury, 1982).

I began to take on a new family role of caregiver for my mother. This began slowly, with flurries of activity. We would visit and help renovate a dilapidated portion of her house. She would call and say that her electricity had been shut off, or that she had no propane to heat her home in the middle of the winter. On one visit, I realized that all the food in her refrigerator was spoiled. As we expressed concern, she would slip deeper into denial.

After difficult contemplation, at a turning point in my personal life, I decided to move my family into her home to help care for her more directly. She was elated for the company and reassured over the assistance and support. Taking on the role of her primary caregiver allowed me to see first-hand the progression of her disease symptoms. It was shocking to see the functional decline and behavioral changes. Much of the role of a caregiver for a person living with Alzheimer's disease involves assisting with activities of daily living (ADL), addressing instrumental needs, as well as navigating behavior changes (i.e., aggression, anger, depression, anxiety, confusion, memory loss, wandering, etc.) at different stages (AA, 2018a; CDC, 2018). We saw each of these depicted over the years of caring for her.

In her working years, my mother was once the food service director for the public school in our community. She always had a passion for culinary arts and food service. At one point in life, she had hoped to start a catering business. But this dream never materialized. Many of her professional goals were set aside to raise and care for us as a single mother. As I reflect upon this, I see the intergenerational reciprocity (Bang, Zhou Koval, & Wade-Benzoni, 2017) that was in motion in our interwoven lives. While I did not realize it at the time, I set aside my professional pursuits to return to my childhood roots and care for her.

Reciprocity applied in this context is the mutually dependent interaction of awareness, attention, and empathy by one to another's (i.e., a parent to their child) needs and perspectives, which in turn develops an awareness, attention, and empathy in the child to the parent's perspective and needs (Sorkhabi, 2012). Reciprocity is inherent in the creation and maintenance of a culture of care within families. The familial culture, established through multiple generations throughout the life course, creates or negates the foundation for a culture of care within the family. Expectations for receiving and providing care are a part of ongoing relationships between family members (Hareven, 2001).

Reciprocity is rooted in generativity. Generativity, the desire and need to invest in other generations, influences family members' views on social roles and social capital, and in turn impacts reciprocity (Hareven, 2001). Attitudes toward generativity are developed by social and relational experiences, which develop values of familial care over the life course (Hareven, 2001).

Since I had returned to my childhood home to care for my mother where she had desired to remain, my son was enrolled in the same school district that I had once been in. Seeing that the moments were slipping away, one day I planned to take my mother to school to have lunch with her grandson. This would mean that she would be returning to the place where she had once worked. I had hoped the experience might stimulate some positive memories from that era of her life. As she was preparing to leave the house, she attempted to style her hair. I realized that she could no longer remember how to do this. She attempted this, refusing assistance, for more than an hour. As I saw her struggle and finally surrender in frustration, my heart sank. Seeing my mother, who was once meticulous about her appearance, no longer able to care for her physical self, was an expression of loss of yet another layer of her former identity.

When we arrived at the school lunchroom, I was able to capture some special photographs with my son and mother. Our visit was short. The sounds, lights, and flurry of activity were so overwhelming for her that she slowly collapsed on the table. I quickly took her out of the room and, as soon as we were away from the overstimulation of the lunchroom, she recovered. There was no discussion of her time working there. No reminiscent memories were recalled. The day was full of many losses, including acknowledging the loss of the long-term memory of her years of working there.

As my mother's disease symptoms progressed over the years, we did all we could to enable her to stay in her home. Seeing the stages of her disease progression was disheartening. She began having frequent extreme emotional outbursts, wandering, and hallucinations. Over the course of four years, we realized that we were reaching the limits of our ability to care for her in her home. We began the daunting task of exploring options for the next phase of her care.

Feeling frustrated much of the time, I felt pulled in too many directions. I was balancing the multigenerational roles of caregiver, wife, and mother, all while working outside of the home. I found very few sources of support, and the ones I did find were very limited.

The role of the "sick" is shared by family and friends whom healthcare clinicians meet, yet it is often only the patient that receives the affordances of illness (Iannarino, 2018). The impact of the illness is experienced by people who are close to the sick, but these supporters, family members, and caregivers are often not recognized (Iannarino, 2018; Odets, 1995). Close supporters also experience biographical disruption, just as patients do. In the case of experiences of supporters, their biographical disruption can be unexpected, burdensome, and is often invisible to others (Odets, 1995). This biographical interdependence is evident in the negotiation and maintenance of support roles. The support role carries feelings of uncertainty, distress, and frustration; yet must continue family, career, and relationship maintenance while also providing support to the patient (Iannarino, 2018).

By 2015 I was at the end of my rope, so we finally started in-home care four days a week. My mother objected, of course, but eventually grew to care deeply for her aide, who was close in age to her and provided both ADL support and companionship. I wish we had started this much sooner. Rose, her in-home care aide, helped care for my mother for less than a year. We soon realized she needed twenty-four-hour care and that our lives were at yet another challenging turning point.

As this reality became salient, I realized I needed all the support I could get for the next steps. I planned a series of family conversations with my brother and our spouses. We visited multiple care facilities in the geographic region. We talked through every possible scenario of breaking the news to our mother, transitioning her there, and her immediate material and care needs. We also addressed end-of-life decisions based on the desires she had expressed in her healthy years.

These family discussions brought up many of our own beliefs and requests, which we shared in varying degrees with each other. We used an interpersonal communication tool in the form of a board game. My Gift of Grace is a "game" designed to facilitate and encourage communication within families about these imperative advance care planning decisions (Van Scoy et al., 2016). There are other resources available to prompt families to share advance care desires. A few are the Five Wishes (Eckstein & Mullener, 2010) and The Conversation Project (Bisognano & Goodman, 2013).

Family conversations could be planned and started as a purposeful measure to share desires and create end-of-life narratives. Pre-need family discussions can open a dialogue during healthy years. Advanced care planning can allow families to focus on interpersonal and relationship related activities and conversations during end-of-life transitions. Family members have an opportunity to share their end-of-life legacies in advance care planning. This allows for families to foster endowments of family legacy.

After our collective sharing of hopes for our own end-of-life narratives, in the following days of 2015, my son who was under the age of ten, began sharing some of his own desires for his life legacy. At a time overwhelmed by so much heaviness and sorrow, I was amazed by these moments of generativity and hope. While I did not find social support in places that I had anticipated, in the way I had hoped (i.e., healthcare providers, support groups, social workers, long-term care facility staff, etc.), I found emotional, esteem, instrumental, and relational support in family, friends, and coworkers (Goldsmith, 2004).

I found solace and healing in writing the story of my caregiving experience. This narrative process has unfolded in many ways and over several years. I hope that it continues throughout my life course journey and into my narrative legacy for future generations. Like others, storytelling was introduced to me through my family.

On my eleventh birthday, I gathered with a few friends at a pizza restaurant. Suddenly, a man jumped into our corner booth and, without introduction, began telling us a story. I looked up at my mother, across the room, and she gave a reassuring nod. I blushed with embarrassment, smiled, and listened in. I have no recollection of what the story was that he told us, but I realized later that my mother had hired a storyteller for my birthday party entertainment. In my early childhood years, I would stay with my grandparents while my mother would work late night shifts waitressing. Night after night, my grandmother would tuck my brother and me in by telling us stories until we drifted off to dream. Perhaps this is where my love of narrative began.

We understand others and ourselves through narrative. We make sense of experiences, form and claim identity, begin our own narratives, and participate in culture through storytelling (Ballard & Ballard, 2011; Langellier & Peterson, 2004). Meaning is constructed and co-constructed partly through narration. Memorable stories are those that resonate with individual, societal, and cultural ideologies and values (Langellier & Peterson, 2004). These stories create reality as it is perceived on a personal, family, cultural, and societal level. As individuals go through an unusual or disruptive experience, their narrative must be reconstructed to understand their identity in reference of the new and the previous contexts. Narrative reconstruction provides a way to reaffirm self-concept and purpose (Williams, 1984).

In the last of her healthy years, my mother began collecting and reading fiction books. At the onset and even as her disease symptoms worsened, she kept on reading. She would read and reread books multiple times. She began writing in the cover the date she read each book. Although she would adamantly deny any memory impairment, she would often laugh and say, "After a while, I forget what the book says, so I just start all over. It's like reading a brand-new story." Some of her books had almost half a dozen dates written in them.

I could get lost in the "I wish things would have been different" woes, but one special narrative experience that I would have liked to have shared with my mother is a book club of sorts. One fascinating family narrative journey is told in the *End of Your Life Book Club* (Schwalbe, 2012). It is a nonfiction auto-ethnographic novel about a woman diagnosed with terminal cancer and her adult son who starts a book club, which strengthens their interpersonal relationship through family communication. Through the experience of participating in a shared activity, the two engage in deep conversations about family, personal, health issues.

While I did not get to experience this with Mom, now I find myself getting lost in a book and smiling, thinking of how my mother *would* have loved the story also. My son is a self-declared "lover of conversation" who shares his daily and ongoing adventure stories. I see that an appreciation of narrative has endured into yet another generation.

After my brother and I finalized the plans to transition my mother to a care facility in 2016 with a specialized dementia care unit, we carefully planned the timing and logistics, finding comfort in the small pieces of the story about which we could manage our uncertainty. In the days before and the week of my mother's move, we adorned her room with family photos of the multiple generations of her family: her parents, siblings, children, and grandchildren. We shared stories with the care staff of her family life and professional adventures.

While the role of primary caregiver was a complex experience full of hardship and rewards, I did not anticipate that it would be so difficult to renegotiate this role as she transitioned to the care facility. It was heartbreaking to see her leave her home and hard to see others caring for her, doing what I could no longer do. Yet it was also comforting knowing that they could care for her in ways that I could not. They offered a level of care that was beyond what we could do at home. While it took some time for adjustment, her needs were being met and she was automatically set in a community of new friends and companions.

As we went through her home in June 2016, packing and sorting her personal items, we discovered many of her things tucked away. In her hidden treasures, I found a journal that she had started in 2010, unbeknownst to us. The cover read "A Mother's Legacy Journal." As I cracked open the pages, it was breathtaking to see her beautiful handwriting that had been stolen away from her, and to read the notes and stories she left us.

She wrote about her childhood, youth, and young adulthood. She shared stories on the pages, some I was very familiar with, some that I was surprised to read. Her stories were interwoven with responses to question prompts. What was your childhood nickname? Who was your first crush? What have you always hoped to do that you haven't done yet? These were questions that I never even thought to ask her. This legacy journal is a priceless treasure. I read from some of the pages during her memorial service.

One of the ways that narrative has emerged and changed since early communication narrative scholarship (Fisher, 1984) is the concept of narrative performance (Langellier & Peterson, 2004). Everyday life is embodied as performance. Individuals and families create stories by co-performing narrative. Narrative has emerged in ethnographic studies of family communication. Goodall (2006) introduced the idea of narrative inheritance as stories that are passed to us as cultural, contextual, and individual family identities. Family storytelling is a narrative act of family legacy in story inheritance (Ballard & Ballard, 2011).

Alemán and Helfrich (2010) introduce narrative inheritance with their research on families experiencing the progressive disease of dementia. Not only is narrative inheritance a process of uncovering and interpreting family narratives, but also an opportunity to create individual stories from family health narratives. Narrative inheritance allows for "insight into the manner in which themes of loss, denial, anxiety, appearance, and care complexly weave through our experiences with dementia" (Alemán & Helfrich, 2010, p. 7). As biological and genetic elements are passed along through birth, children inherit physiological qualities of their ancestors. Stories are also passed along. Descendants experience genetic and narrative inheritance but also are writing unique narratives of their own.

Ballard and Ballard (2011) introduce a shift from narrative inheritance into joint family creation of stories as narrative momentum, which focuses on the sense of movement in narrative and the force that carries families into the future. Family legacy as well as genetic health concerns present opportunities for individuals and families to use narrative momentum to write their own stories of new traditions, values, and health decisions.

I contrasted my mother's legacy journal stories to those in the last years of her life. So much of the narrative of her last years of life included confusion and loss. How could she have forgotten where her red hair came from (i.e., her father)? How could she have forgotten who her son was, or that her brother had died decades earlier? Like many other dementia sufferers, she was at times lost in the waves of mental anguish. As we saw the horrors of confusion and unusual behavior, we relayed these stories to health professionals, attempting to convey her mounting needs through narrative.

Other times, as she was calm and at peace, experiencing an alternate reality, we met her there by performing narrative. We saw the dementia professionals caring for Mom use this mode of compassionate treatment and care by stepping into the narrative she was experiencing at that moment. Our family had to face a new approach to narrative. No longer did the strict tenets of probability and fidelity apply (Fisher, 1984). This experience is not unique. Millions of other families are experiencing a similar journey of loss, denial, anxiety, and care complexity across multiple generations (AA, 2018b).

Families facing this difficult illness journey can partner with health providers to both individually and collectively enact narrative; to bear witness to experiences of dementia caregiving and relational navigation. As storytellers, we

> cannot turn from the sufferings of [our] characters. A storyteller, unlike a historian, must follow compassion wherever it leads . . . [and] accompany characters, even into smoke and fire, and bear witness to what they thought and felt even when they themselves no longer knew. (Maclean, 1992, p. 102)

Health professionals cared for my mother for eighteen months between 2016 and 2017 in the dementia facility. Alzheimer's is a slow, progressive disease (CDC, 2018). There is currently no cure. Family members can experience an intense sense of loss and grief, even in the absence of death, as the patient slowly declines (Pearlin, 2010). Our grief began long before she died. It continues still.

In her last six months of life, as hospice care began in the summer of 2017, we knew the time was drawing near. She lost her ability to verbally communicate in the last months. We painfully watched the disease slowly consume the last of her body's physical functioning. My brother and I gathered to be next to her the last ten days of her life. As our hearts broke, we stayed awake several nights at her bedside and comforted each other with recounted childhood stories.

We were there with her as she drew her last breath on October 28, 2017. We felt the weight of overwhelming loss, having slowly lost the last years with her. Grief is strange and funny. When I sit down with intentions to engage in "grieving," it is often fruitless. Yet, when for example a catalog arrives in the mail selling vintage ceramic Christmas trees just like the one my mother had, the feelings of grief can hit me out of nowhere. It can also bombard me from the storyline of a film. I recently watched the movie *Wit*, which tells the story of an English professor diagnosed with stage-four cancer (Bosanquet & Nichols, 2001). I was not anticipating this to evoke so many of the memories of my personal experience watching my mother, from her bedside, as her body slowly slipped from life into death. She was unconscious for most of the time during her last two weeks of life. In the film, a similar situation is depicted. The nurse rubs lotion onto her unconscious patient's arms, similar to the ways that the staff lovingly cared for my mother. They would, as depicted in the film, talk softly and compassionately to my mother even though she was sleeping soundly. They very gently repositioned her, swabbed her mouth, changed her clothes, and rubbed warm lotion on her arms and legs. The most profound experience etched into the narrative of my memory of my mother's dying was watching them wash and care for her body immediately after she passed away. When I reflect on these moments, I do not see loss and death. Instead I see the compassion and beauty of the human experience, when we care for one another in our most vulnerable states.

We long for these experiences. We long for companionship and relationship. This is echoed in much communication research. One exemplar is Cole, Kemeny, and Taylor (1997), who note that social rejection and isolation have devastating psychological and physical implications. Narrative invites us together. We understand our experiences, ourselves, and our relationships through narrative (Langellier & Peterson, 2004). Relationships are cultivated by stories.

Health, family, and lifespan communication scholars must continue extending narrative scholarship. Families can find hope within an experience of dementia by utilizing narrative momentum to write their own stories of new traditions, values, and health decisions (Ballard & Ballard, 2011). Additionally, persons diagnosed with dementia and their family members can implement narrative reconstruction to redefine self-concept and reaffirm purpose (Nelson, 2001; Williams, 1984).

Narrative can improve health experiences and familial relationships. A new trajectory for narrative scholarship must embrace the fragmented stories of persons living with dementia (Steeman, Tournoy, Grypdonck, Godderis, & De Casterlé, 2013), and the fragmented collection of health narratives as layered, multigenerational, collective accounts. As family members seek social support, create community, and develop culture, the legacy of their stories will ignite passion for others to share and create their own narratives. Familial caregivers and health professionals can share narratives of experience and interaction for education and support. This narrative contagion can create opportunities for better health and stronger families.

Healthcare professionals can better serve patients and their family members with narrative medicine (Charon, 2006) and narrative palliative care (Stanley & Hurst, 2011). Narrative is not only a means of practicing empathy and enhancing care. Narrative can also be a means of self-reflection and growth for health professionals as they make sense of their identities as clinicians and their experiences caring for patients (Kalitzkus & Matthiessen,

2009). Narrative is an enlightening means of understanding and sensemaking into the nature of medicine and human experience.

Frank (1998) conceptualizes illness narratives as taking on three forms. One is a restitution story. This is a story of restored health. The heroes defeat the enemy of disease. The restitution story is what is preferred. We hope to live on and maintain health. The second type is the chaos story. This is the most feared. It is full of uncertainty and anxiety. When we hear others' stories of uncertainty, we think, "That could happen to anyone. That could happen to me." The last variety is the quest story. In this type of illness narrative, the experience of illness leads to new insights. We form new components of self-identity. A quest story requires letting go of the old qualities of one's self (Frank, 1998).

We all will experience illness in some form throughout the life course. What story will your family write? What types of stories will you share? My hope is that we embrace the narratives we inherit and continue writing and sharing our stories for living, dying, and leaving a legacy to future generations. We cannot all anticipate experiencing restitution stories. However, we all can come to see our lives as quest stories.

REFERENCES

Alemán, M. W., & Helfrich, K. W. (2010). Inheriting the narratives of dementia: A collaborative tale of a daughter and mother. *Journal of Family Communication, 10,* 7–23. doi:10.1080/15267430903385784.

Alzheimer's Association. (2018a). *Stages and behaviors.* Retrieved from https://www.alz.org/help-support/caregiving/stages-behaviors.

Alzheimer's Association. (2018b). *2018 Alzheimer's disease facts and figures.* Retrieved from http://www.alz.org/facts/overview.asp.

Ballard, R. L., & Ballard, S. J. (2011). From narrative inheritance to narrative momentum: Past, present, and future stories in an international adoptive family. *Journal of Family Communication, 11,* 69–84. doi:10.1080/15267431.2011.554618.

Bang, H. M., Zhou Koval, C., & Wade-Benzoni, K. A. (2017). It's the thought that counts over time: The interplay of intent, outcome, stewardship, and legacy motivations in intergenerational reciprocity. *Journal of Experimental Social Psychology, 73*(1), 197–210.

Belk, R. W. (1988). Possessions and the extended self. *Journal of Consumer Research, 15*(2), 139–168.

Bisognano, M., & Goodman, E. (2013). Engaging patients and their loved ones in the ultimate conversation. *Health Affairs, 32,* 203–206. doi:10.1377/hlthaff.2012.1174.

Bosanquet, S. (Producer) & Nichols, M. (Director). (2001). *Wit* [Motion picture]. United States: HBO Films and Avenue Pictures.

Bury, M. (1982). Chronic illness as biographical disruption. *Sociology of Health and Illness, 4,* 167–182.

Centers for Disease Control and Prevention. (2018). *Alzheimer's disease.* Retrieved from https://www.cdc.gov/aging/aginginfo/alzheimers.htm.

Charmaz, K. (1999). From the "sick role" to stories of self: Understanding the self in illness. In R. J. Contrada & R. D. Ashmore (Eds.), *Self, social identity, and physical health: Interdisciplinary explorations* (pp. 209–239). New York: Oxford University Press.

Charon, R. (2006). *Narrative medicine: Honoring the stories of illness.* New York: Oxford University Press.

Cole, S. W., Kemeny, M. E., & Taylor, S. E. (1997). Social identity and physical health: Accelerated HIV progression in rejection-sensitive gay men. *Journal of Personality and Social Psychology, 72*, 320–335.

Eckstein, D., & Mullener, B. (2010). A couples advance directives interview using the Five Wishes questionnaire. *The Family Journal: Counseling and Therapy for Couples and Families, 18*, 66–69. doi: 10.1177/1066480709357748.

Elder, G. H. (1998). The life course as development theory. *Child Development, 69*(1), 1–12.

Fisher, W. R. (1984). Narration as a human communication paradigm: The case of public moral argument. *Communication Monographs, 51*, 1–22. doi:10.1080/03637758409390180

Frank, A. W. (1998). Just listening: Narrative and deep illness. *Families, Systems, and Health, 16*, 197–212.

Goldsmith, D. J. (2004). *Communicating social support.* New York: Cambridge University Press.

Goodall, H. (2006). Why we must win the war on terror. *Qualitative Inquiry, 12*(1), 30–59.

Greenfield, E., Oberlink, M., Scharlach, A., Neal, M., & Stafford, P. (2015). Age-friendly community initiatives: Conceptual issues and key questions. *The Gerontologist, 55*(2), 191–198.

Hareven, T. K. (2001). Historical perspectives on aging and family relations. In Robert H. Binstock & L. K. George (Eds.), *Handbook of aging and the social sciences* (5th ed., pp. 141–159). San Diego, CA: Academic Press.

Iannarino, N. T. (2018). "It's my job now, I guess": Biographical disruption and communication work in supporters of young adult cancer survivors. *Communication Monographs*, 1–24. doi:10.1080/03637751.2018.1468916

Kalitzkus, V., & Matthiessen, P. F. (2009). Narrative-based medicine: Potential, pitfalls, and practice. *The Permanente Journal, 13*, 80–86.

Karp, D. (1997). *Speaking of sadness.* Oxford: Oxford University Press.

Langellier, K. M. & Peterson, E. E. (2004). *Storytelling in daily life: Performing narrative.* Philadelphia, PA: Temple University Press.

Maclean, N. (1992). *Young men and fire*, p. 102. Chicago: University of Chicago Press.

Mittal, B. (2006). I, me, and mine-how products become consumers' extended selves. *Journal of Consumer Behaviour, 5*(6), 550–562.

Nelson, H. (2001). *Damaged identities, narrative repair.* Ithaca: Cornell University Press.

Odets, W. (1995). *In the shadow of the epidemic: Being HIV negative in the age of AIDS.* Durham, NC: Duke University Press.

Parsons, T. (1951). *The social system.* Glencoe, IL: The Free Press.

Pearlin, L. I. (2010). The life course and the stress process: Some conceptual comparisons. *Journal of Gerontology: Social Sciences, 65B*(2), 207–215. doi:10.1093/geronb/gbp106.

Pound, P., Gompertz, P., & Ebrahim, S. (1998). Illness in the context of older age: The case of stroke. *Sociology of Health and Illness, 20*, 489–506.

Proshansky, H. M., Fabian, A. K., & Kaminoff, R. (1983). Place-identity: Physical world socialization of the self. *Journal of Environmental Psychology, 3*(1), 57–83.

Satariano, W., Scharlach, A., & Lindeman, D. (2014). Aging, place, and technology: Toward improving access and wellness in older populations. *Journal of Aging and Health, 26*(8), 1373–1389.

Schwalbe, W. (2012). *The end of your life book club.* New York: Alfred A. Knopf, Random House.

Sorkhabi, N. (2012). Parent socialization effects in different cultures: Significance of directive parenting. *Psychological Reports, 110*(3), 854–878.

Stanley, P., & Hurst, M. (2011). Narrative palliative care: A method for building empathy. *Journal of Social Work in End-of-Life & Palliative Care, 7*, 39–55. doi:10.1080/15524256.2011.548046

Steeman, E., Tournoy, J., Grypdonck, M., Godderis, J., & De Casterlé, B. D. (2013). Managing identity in early-stage dementia: Maintaining a sense of being valued. *Ageing and Society, 33*(2), 216–242.

Van Scoy, L. J., Scott, A. M., Reading, J. M., Chuang, C. H., Chinchilli, V. M., Levi, B. H., & Green, M. J. (2016). From theory to practice: Measuring end-of-life communication quality using multiple goals theory. *Patient Education and Counseling, 100*(5), 1–10. doi:10.1016/j.pec.2016.12.010.

Vignoles, V. L., Schwartz S. J., Luyckx, K. (2011). Introduction: Toward an integrative view of identity. In: Schwartz S., Luyckx K., Vignoles V. (Eds) *Handbook of identity theory and research* (pp. 1–24). New York: Springer.

Williams, G. (1984). The genesis of chronic illness: narrative re-construction. *Sociology of Health & Illness, 6*(2), 175–200.

Index

abdominal pain, 109
abscess, 77
activist, 87
activities of daily living (ADLs), 203
addiction, cigarette, 75, 76–77
ADLs. *See* activities of daily living
adults, older, 156, 168, 190, 202
Advair, 78
advanced directives, 184
advocate, 4; patient, 76, 177
"ages and stages" approach, 1
aggression, 203
aging, 156, 190, 202
agitation, 140
aides, home health, 85
allergens, desensitization to, 55–57
allergen statement, 48
allergic reactions, 43–44, 53
allergies, 4, 82; accommodations for, 49, 52; anaphylaxis and, 43–44, 53; antibiotic use and, 45; classroom policy for, 55; food, 43–57; hives, 43; limitations with, 47; peanut, 43, 44, 47, 48, 56; POCHA group, 49; protocol for, 54; risk for developing, 44; testing for, 50–51, 53–54, 56. *See also* specific allergies
allergist, 48, 53, 55, 57
almonds, 48, 56
Alzheimer's disease, 5–6, 201, 203, 209; dominantly inherited, 139, 140, 148; early onset, 139–148; family history of, 142; managing interpersonal relationships and, 139–148; research and awareness for, 147, 147–148
Alzheimer's narrative: collecting and writing, 140–148; family history, 142; future plans, 146–148; importance of family, 142–144; method, 141–142; relationships, 146; until Alzheimer's do us Part, 144–145
American Cancer Society, 68
amniotic fluid, 16
amyloid plaques, 140, 148
amyloid precursor protein (APP) genes, 140, 148
amyloid-β peptides, 140
anaphylaxis, 43–44, 53
anesthesia, 155
anesthesiologist, 16, 17, 64, 153, 155, 165
anger, 29, 203
antibiotic use, 46; allergies and, 45
anxiety, 114, 115, 123, 153, 203, 208; panic attacks and, 159, 160
aortic stenosis (AS), 156, 157, 170n5
apnea, 12, 131
APP. *See* amyloid precursor protein genes
arthritis, 176
AS. *See* aortic stenosis
assisted living, 196
assumptions, 156, 192
asthma, 4, 78, 80, 198

audiogram, 103
audiologist, 97, 102, 103
audiology, 103, 105
audiometry booth, 102
auricle, 103
autoethnographic narrative, 25–26, 109–119
autoethnography, 122; personal experiences and, 110–112
autonomy, 167, 178–179
autopsy, 142

barriers, cultural and language, 37, 126
bedrest, 13–14
Beethoven, 103
behavior, changes in, 203
behind the ear (BTE) hearing aids, 108
Beowulf, 100–102
biographical disruptions, 203, 205
biomedical explanations, 2
birth, 3–4, 10–11, 109; breech, 77; C-section, 16, 17, 19, 31; experiences, 16–18; of multiples, 12, 15; premature, 11–12, 11–20, 69; in unfamiliar environment, 25–40; weight, 69
birth narrative: far from home, 29; communicating without language, 31–32; course of action, 38–39; delivery and birth, 16–18; discussion of, 20–21; fear of losing baby, 30–31; forming new relationships, 35–36; high-risk and premature; maintaining positivity, 33–34; method, 12–13; need for personal self-examination, 37–38; neonatal experiences, 18–20; new survivor self-identity, 36–37; open at every stage, 34–35; pregnancy experience, 13–16; recommendations, 37–39; social media, 34–35; social support and coping, 39–40
bladder, 112; condition of, 109–110; control of, 81; leakage, 117; medication for, 114; spasms, 110
blood pressure: high, 12, 160; lowered, 43; preeclampsia and, 12, 15
body: control of, 115, 116, 117, 119; wasting, 140
bone: spurs, 177; strength, 124
bony labyrinth, 103

brain: bleed, 12; damage, 12; degeneration, 139, 140
Brazil nuts, 56
breastfeeding, 44
bronchitis, 78
Bruss, Kasey, 4
BTE. *See* behind the ear hearing aids

Calvin, Krista, 32, 36, 38
cancer, 122; American Cancer Society, 68; of breast, 124; chemotherapy for, 61, 64, 65, 66, 129, 176; in childhood, 61; colorectal, 124; endometrial, 124; of kidney, 61, 63; non-Hodgkin's lymphoma, 176; ovarian, 124; overcoming, 175; prostate, 196; radiation for, 61, 64, 68, 176, 177; stage-four, 209; survivor, 61, 62, 63, 65–67, 124, 129, 134, 174; terminal, 207; treatments, 68
care: communal, 167; communication of, 158–160; end of life, 209–210
caregiver: caring for, 6; for family, 162, 203; feedback of, 40; long distance, 158, 160, 170; outside, 166; personhood of, 154; primary, 158, 207; sister as, 143; spouse as, 142; viewpoint of, 3
caregiving, 158–160, 169; dementia and, 209; for family, 6, 162; at home, 158, 178; shifting roles in, 160
caretaker. *See* caregiver
cashews, 48, 56
CAT. *See* communication accommodation theory
cataracts, 78
cerebral palsy, 12
certified management accountant (CMA), 189
certified public accountant (CPA), 189
cervix, incompetent, 12
cesarean sections (C-section), 16; emergency, 17, 19, 31. *See also* birth
change: accepting, 124; in behavior, 203; in diet, 123; in emotions, 122; in end of life conversations, 193–195; navigating, 193–195; openness to, 28; in personality, 140; stability and, 177–178
chaos story, 211

Charon, Rita, 139
chemotherapy, 61, 64, 65, 66, 129, 176. *See also* cancer
chest pain, 121
childbirth, 10–11, 109. *See also* birth
childhood, 4
chronic condition, 167; coping with, 109–119; inherited, 148; self-management of, 118
chronic illness narrative: college years, 67–68; in-between and onset of survivor guilt, 65–67; reflection, 71–72; start of it all, 63–65; the unknown, 68–71
chronic obstructive pulmonary disease (COPD), 79, 80, 83
cigarettes, 75, 76–77. *See also* smoking
classrooms, allergy policy for, 55
clinical trials, 143, 147
CMA. *See* certified management accountant
Cobb, Jamie, 5
cochlea, 103
cochlear implants, 108
cognitive abilities, 195
cognitive impairment, 140
collaborative interviewing, 141
coma, medical, 155, 165
communal support, 140, 148
communication: agency, 161–164; of care, 158–160; direct, 185; doctor-patient, 76, 129; effectiveness of, 126; empathic, 76; end-of-life, 184; in family, 208; gerontology research on, 157; of health and disability, 75, 154; without language, 31–32; language barriers in, 30; lifespan and health, 1, 166–167, 167, 169, 210; loss of, 140; narrative as, 9; native languages, 129; ongoing, 184; physician, 184; positive, 88, 174–175; process of, 5; relational, 5, 6; research, 163, 166–167, 210; studying, 161, 174; supportive, 25; translator for, 30
communication accommodation theory (CAT), 190, 192
communication theory of identity, 192
communicative phenomena, 26
companionship, 159, 166, 210

compassion, 186
confusion, 202, 203
connectedness, autonomy and, 178–179
connection, narrative for, 11
constipation, 117
control, lack of, 114
convergence, 190
conversations: CAT, 190; end of life, 189–198; family, 205; father-daughter, 189–198; final, 185–186
Cooks, Leda, 5
COPD. *See* chronic obstructive pulmonary disease
coping, 26, 34, 39–40, 62, 111; abilities, 118; communal, 143; strategies, 123
CPA. *See* certified public accountant
C-section. *See* cesarean sections
culture, 5, 27, 28, 32, 110, 122–123; healthcare and, 134–135; pregnancy and, 10
cystitis. *See* interstitial cystitis, living with

day care, 49, 51
deafness, 5, 94, 102; analogy for, 105, 107; belonging and, 104; connection to, 106; culture of, 106; meaning to, 106; medical side of, 104; metaphors for, 108; raising children in, 107–108; silence and, 106; story of, 103
death, 29, 83
decision making, 9
delivery: emergency, 16, 17; experiences, 16–18
dementia, 139, 147, 194, 207, 208, 210; caregiving for, 209
Demerol, 78
dental complications, 77–78
dependence, 167, 196
depression, 66, 123, 131, 132, 203; in menopause, 123
dermatologist, 195; pediatric, 46
diabetes, 12
diagnosis, with meaning, 93–108
dialectic tensions, 175–176
dialogic complexity, 176
dialogue, 110
diet change, 123
disability, 4; ownership of, 106; physical and emotional demands of, 76

disclosure to others, 28
discrimination, 52
disease: chronic, 62; living with, 75; progressive, 84; terminal, 84
disruptions and illnesses: chronic, 3, 4; health, 1; narratives of, 9–10; struggles and adaptations to, 4
dissociation, during birth, 29
divergence, 190
diverticulosis, 176
doctor, native language with, 129
Dominantly Inherited Alzheimer's Disease, 139, 140, 148
dynamics, relational, 2

ear, 50, 102
early onset Alzheimer's disease, 139–148. *See also* Alzheimer's disease
Easy Lift, 178–179, 179–180, 181
eczema, 77
eggs, 43
elderly, 168, 202. *See also* adults
electrocardiogram, 121
emotions, 4, 110; challenges with, 122; changes in, 122; extreme, 147; outbursts of, 202; support for, 132–133, 134, 145
emphysema, 4, 78
empowerment, 3, 125–126
encounters, public and private, 179–181
end of life conversations narrative, 189–193; navigating changes in, 193–195; new identity in, 195–196; patienthood needs in, 196; role reversal in, 197–198
End of Your Life Book Club, 207
endometriosis, 112
endometritis, 129
English as a second language (ESL), 126, 130, 134–135
"enmeshed in narrative", 2
environment, 123
epinephrine, 43–44
Epi-Pen injector, 48, 49
escape-denial, 67
ESL. *See* English as a second language
exercise, aerobic, 124–125
expectations: during high-risk pregnancy and premature birth, 9–21; reality and, 17, 20–21
experiences: autoethnography and, 110–112; delivery and birth, 16–18; drawing from, 2; emotional, 25; of hardship, 28; of illness and disability, 111; mental, 25; near-death, 28; neonatal, 18–20; physical, 25; pregnancy, 13–16; therapeutic, 111; transformative, 27–29

fallopian tubes, 112
family caregiving narrative, 201–211
family leave, after birth, 45
family relationships, 142–144
fatigue, 123, 131
fear, 167; of losing baby, 30–31
feelings, 71–72
fertility, 13, 112
fetal distress, 12
fetal movement, 15–16
financial planner, 146
financial stability, 147
fish, 43
Flonase, 96, 97
food allergens, 43; rates of, 49
food allergies: genetics and, 45; immune system and, 43; management protocol for, 54; narrative of, 43–57; navigating, 43–57; outgrowing, 53. *See also* allergies
food allergy narrative: finding our way, 49–52; first diagnosis, 47–49; professor, mother, and patient, 44–45; public school, 54–55; searching for answers, 45–47; turning the tide, 55–57; a way of life, 52–54
foreign environment, 25–26. *See also* birth narrative, far from home
Fox-Hines, Ruthann, 4
fractures, 124
fragility, resilience and, 181–187
frames of reference, 192, 193
Frankl, Victor, 29
friendships, 146
future: after cancer, 68–71; framing of, 165; uncertain, 147

genetic mutation, 143, 148
genetics, 123; food allergies and, 45

genetic screening, 140
genetic testing, 142, 148
gerontology research, 157, 161, 202
Gilbert, Melissa, 103
glass, darkly through, 93–108
glaucoma, 78
gratitude, 198
grief, 13, 14, 209
guilt, of survivor, 61, 65–67
gymnastics, 65
gynecologist, 79

hair loss, 64
Hall, Jennifer, 4
hand washing, 55
healing, narrative for, 11
health care, culturally appropriate, 134–135
health communication. *See* communication
health disruptions, illnesses and, 1, 3
health insurance, long-term, 146
health narrative approach, 26–27; transformative experiences, 27–29. *See also* narrative
hearing: aids, 99–100, 102, 103, 105, 106, 108; lipreading and, 107; loss of, 12, 99, 102, 103, 107; ReSound, 105; test, 97, 99
heart: attack, 121, 122; conditions, 12, 122; disease, 121; failure, 169; valve replacement, 156
heightened sensitivity to life, 28
HELPP syndrome, 12
hematoma, 129
hemorrhage, 129
Heston, Charlton, 147
hippocampus, 140
hives, 43
home health services, 85
Hope-Gill, Laura, 5
hormone replacement therapy, 124
hormones, 79; treatment with, 122, 124–125
hospice care, 186, 209
hot flushes, 122, 131
humiliation, 112
hyperthyroid, 132
hysterectomy, 129, 176

IC. *See* interstitial cystitis
ICU. *See* intensive care unit
identity, 167, 201; communication theory of, 192; crisis, 65; dynamic, 193; former, 204; gap, 195; impacts on, 202; new, 190; perceptions of, 164; reconstructing new, 195–196; shifting, 178; threats, 115
IgE. *See* immunoglobulin E
illness, chronic, 61–72
immune response, 53; desensitizing, 56
immune system, 80; food allergies and, 43; immature, 12
immunoglobulin E (IgE), 53
inanition, 140
independence, 195–196, 202
individualism, 161, 167
infection, 12, 164
infertility, 13
information, access to, 125
inquiry: appreciative, 168; process of, 110
insensitivity, of medical providers, 75
instinct, protective, 57
insurance, 146, 168
intensive care unit (ICU), 153, 155
interaction, 163
interpersonal relationships, Alzheimer's disease and, 139–148
interstitial cystitis (IC), 5; living with, 109–119; management of, 118; medication for, 114; treatment for, 115–117
interstitial cystitis (IC) narrative: health status, 112; hope on horizon, 115–118; introduction, 112–114; living in harmony, 118–119; ruling life, 114–115
interview guide, 142
intrauterine growth restriction (IUGR), 12
iron deficiency anemia, 123
isolation, 87, 210; illness and, 85; risk for, 88; social, 89n2
IUGR. *See* intrauterine growth restriction

jaundice, 12

Keller, Helen, 103
kidney: cancer, 61, 63; disease, 61, 68, 70; failing, 185
Kratzer, Jessica M. W., 5

labor: premature, 10, 12; in unfamiliar environment, 25–40
legacy: of family caregiving, 201–211; leaving, 211; life, 206; "A Mother's Legacy Journal", 207–208
life: after health disruptions, 71; insurance, 146; legacy, 206; meaning in, 3; quality of, 122–123, 154
lifespan: communication perspective, 61; identity development, 155; narrative perspective, 161; understanding of, 6
life story, 154
linked lives, 173–187
lipreading, 107
listener, 26
listening devices, 99–100, 102
loon, cry of, 93–94, 94–96, 108
lungs: damage to, 75; fluid in, 159
lupus, 100

macadamia nuts, 56
malnutrition, 140
Marcaine, 116, 117
The March of Dimes, 11
massage therapy, 177
maternal age, advanced, 12
McIntyre, Robin, 5, 139–148
media, 11, 13, 18; social, 34–35
medical: jargon, 157; procedures, 10; providers, 75; school, 76
medication: Advair, 78; antibiotics, 45, 46; bladder, 114; Demerol, 78; Marcaine, 116, 117; morphine, 184; pain, 78; sedative, 155; steroids, 78, 79, 83; Xanax, 160
memory, 140; long-term, 204; loss of, 196, 203. *See also* dementia
menopause: chemical-induced, 124; perimenopause disorder, 121, 123, 132; symptoms of, 125; taboo of, 124; themes for ESL in, 128–133
menopause narrative: doctor visits, treatment, and procedures, 129–131; with ESL, 121–135; literature review, 122–123; mood swaying, stress, and complaints, 131–132; social and emotional support, 132–133; theoretical framework and methods, 126–128; wellness, hormones, and exercise in, 124–126
menstrual bleeding, 132
menstrual cycles, end of, 122
mental defeat, 29
mental health, 37, 71, 160
mental retardation, 12
middle-age, 4–5
migration, 123
milk, 43
miscarriage, 69
mood swaying, 131–132
Morey Hawkins, Jennifer, 4
morphine, 184
"A Mother's Legacy Journal", 207–208
motivation, 3
music settings, 102
My Gift of Grace game, 205

narrative: Alzheimer's, 140–148; autoethnographic, 25–26, 109–119; as communication, 9; connection, 11; definition of, 26; differences in, 11; of end of life conversations, 189–198; enmeshed in, 2; exploration, 173–187; of family caregiving, 201–211; father-daughter, 189–198; of food allergies, 43–57; foreclosure, 161–162; of geriatrics, 163; of giving birth far from home, 29–37; of healing, 11; as healing and connection, 11; of health, 3, 26–29, 110–112; health disruptions as, 9–10; of high-risk pregnancy, 11–20; of IC, 112–119; importance of, 3; inheritance, 208; inquiry, 2, 141; lessons from, 166–170; of lifespan, 161; of medicine, 210; of menopause, 121–135; momentum, 208, 210; of older people, 161; of patienthood, 153–170; performance, 208; personal, 3; political, 2; of positivity, 173–187; of pregnancy, 10–20; of pregnancy and childbirth, 10–11; of premature birth, 11–20; relational, 166–170; researchers, 161; response to, 11; sharing, 211; of smoking, 75–88; strategies, 165; theorists, 154; therapeutic effects of, 26–27; understanding others through, 206; of women's health, 1, 2; writing, 2

Narrative Medicine: Honoring the Stories of Illness, 139
narrator, 26
nasal decongestant, 96
nature, 29
ND. *See* nicotine dependency
necrotizing enterocolitis, 12
need for information, 28
neoliberalism, 167
neonatal intensive care unit (NICU), 12–13, 15, 17, 18–20, 21, 31, 33
neurologist, 201, 202
Nicorette Gum, 76
nicotine dependency (ND), 89n1
nicotine gum, 76
NICU. *See* neonatal intensive care unit
noise, 102
non-Hodgkin's lymphoma, 176
norms, societal and cultural, 9
nuts. *See specific nuts*

OIT. *See* oral immunotherapy
openness to change, 28
ophthalmologist, 78
optimism, 174
oral immunotherapy (OIT), 55–57
organ, prolapsed, 112
otologist, 97
otoscope, 98, 99
ovaries, 112
oxygen: dependence on, 75; home, 82, 83–84; levels, 80, 86; portable, 84, 86; power outage and, 84; therapy, 82

pain: abdominal, 109; chest, 121; medication for, 78
panic attacks, 159, 160. *See also* anxiety
parenthood, 196
Parents of Children Who Have Allergies (POCHA) group, 49
Parks, Rosa, 147
Patent Ductus Arteriosus (PDA), 12
patient: advocate, 76, 177; practitioner and, 176–177, 183
patienthood, 25–40; construction of, 154; negotiating, 190
patienthood narrative: communicating agency, 161–164; communicating care as identity, 158–160; continuing story of, 170; miracles in, 164–166; personal and relations in, 153–170; relational, 166–170; Sylvia's story, 153–170
PDA. *See* Patent Ductus Arteriosus
peanut, 43, 44; allergy, 48; butter, 47; flour, 56; protein, 56
pecans, 48, 56
pelvic floor muscles, 114
pelvis, 112
perimenopause disorder, 121, 123, 132. *See also* menopause
periods, irregular, 122
personal growth, 118
personality change, 140
physical therapy, 109, 177
pistachios, 48, 56
placenta previa, 12
pleurodesis, 156, 170n4
pneumonectomy, 156
pneumonia, 80, 140
POCHA. *See* Parents of Children Who Have Allergies group
polycystic ovarian syndrome, 98
positivity, 35; in communication, 88, 174–175; maintaining, 33–34; in patient experience, 173–187
positivity narrative, 173; autonomy and connectedness in, 178–179; change and stability in, 177–178; communication in, 174–175; dialectic tensions in, 175–176; patient and practitioner in, 176–177; public and private encounters in, 179–181; resilience and fragility in, 181–187
postnatal period, 25
posttraumatic growth (PTG), 118–119
post-traumatic stress disorder (PTSD), 66
practitioner, patient and, 176–177, 183
preeclampsia, 12, 15
pregnancy, 3–4; culture and, 10; expectations during, 9–21; experiences, 13–16; high risk, 11–20; narrative of, 10–20
premature rupture of membranes (PROM), 12
prematurity. *See* birth, premature
prenatal care, 10
preschool program, 51, 52–53
presenilin 1 (PSEN1), 140, 148

presenilin 2 (PSEN2), 140, 148
preterm birth. *See* birth, premature
PROM. *See* premature rupture of membranes
PSEN1. *See* presenilin 1
PSEN2. *See* presenilin 2
psychiatrist, 160
psychology, 161
PTG. *See* posttraumatic growth
PTSD. *See* post-traumatic stress disorder
public school, 54–55
pulmonologist, 78
purgatory, 153

quest stories, 211

radiation, 61, 64, 68, 176, 177. *See also* cancer
Randall-Griffiths, Deleasa, 5
RDT. *See* relational dialectics theory
Reagan, Ronald, 147
reality: adapting to, 4; expectations and, 17, 20–21
reciprocity, intergenerational, 203–204
reference, frames of, 192–193
rejection, social, 210
relational dialectics theory (RDT), 175–176
relationships, 160, 169, 210; Alzheimer's disease and, 139–148; embarrassing moments in, 128–129; family, 142–144; far from home, 35–36; interpersonal, 139–148, 207; mother-daughter, 175; new, 35–36; physician-patient, 126; shared experiences, 146
research, 44, 57; health, 202
residence, attachment to, 202
resilience, 88; fragility and, 181–187
ReSound, 105
respect, 168
respiratory disease, smoking and, 75
respiratory distress syndrome, 12
response, empathic, 3
restitution story, 211
restroom, location of, 114
retinopathy of prematurity (ROP), 12
roles: boundaries in, 203; in caregiving, 160; multigenerational, 205; reversal in, 190, 197–198

Ronald and Nancy Reagan Research Institute, 147
root canal, 77
ROP. *See* retinopathy of prematurity
rumination, 29

safety, 25
sarcoma, 66
scar: surgical, 70; tissue, 112
sedative, 155
self-care, 169
self-catheterize, 116, 117
self-communication, 27–28
self-disclosure, 145
self-esteem, 123, 124
self-examination: course of action for, 38–39; personal, 37–38; social support and coping in, 39
self-identity, 28, 40, 211; survivor, 36–37
self-pity, 146
self-reflection, 40, 210
self-transformation, 25–40
self-worth, 117
semicircular canals, 103
sense of coherence (SOC), 161
sensitivity, 36
sensorineural hearing loss, 99
sepsis, 164
sesame seeds, 56
sexism, 156
sexual desire, 124
shellfish, 43
shock, 43
sign language, 107
silence, deafness and, 106
sinus congestion, 96
sleep: apnea, 131; difficulty, 122, 131
smoking, 4, 28; addiction, 75, 76–77; advertisement of, 75; behaviors, 75; cessation of, 125; confronting constraints with, 75–88; damage from, 77; effects of, 78; legacy of, 75–88; narrative, 75–88; ND, 89n1; Nicorette Gum, 76; nicotine gum, 76; resilience and, 88; respiratory disease and, 75; tobacco companies, 75
SOC. *See* sense of coherence
social: constructivism, 26; embarrassments, 128–129; media,

34–36; networking, 31, 35–36; support, 10, 39–40, 124, 126, 132–133, 134, 140, 144, 148
soybeans, 43
speech: delay, 50; therapist, 97
Spencer, Elizabeth A., 6
spleen, 63
sports, contact, 65
stability, change and, 177–178
stereotyping, 156, 191
sternotomy, 153, 157, 170n1
steroids, 78, 79, 83
St. Jude's Children's Research Hospital, 64
stories: chaos, 211; life, 2, 161; as memories, 173; quest, 211; restitution, 211; of Sylvia, 153–170; value of, 11
storytelling, 2–3, 62, 110
stress, 121, 131–132, 134
stroke, 122, 195
Sun, Wei, 5
sunflower seeds, 56
support system, 4, 25, 26, 86, 88, 206; communal, 140, 148; emotional, 36, 132–133, 134, 145; foreign, 35–36; in home, 158, 205; home health, 85; intergenerational, 6; lack of, 109; loss of, 202; online, 35–36; resources, 75; social, 134, 140, 144, 148; spousal, 134
surfactant, 12
surgeon, 153, 156
surgery: emergency, 63–64; open heart, 160
survivor, 165; of cancer, 61, 62, 63, 65–67, 124, 129, 134, 174; guilt, 61, 65–67; self-identity, 36–37
survivorship, 62, 134
swelling, 43

TAVR. *See* transcatheter aortic valve replacement
tensions, 155; dialectic, 175–176
thoracentesis, 159, 170n6
thoracotomy, 156, 170n3
tobacco companies, 75
transcatheter aortic valve replacement (TAVR), 155, 170n2
transcendence, 29
"transcendent experiences", 28
transformation theory, 29

transformative experiences, 31, 32, 34, 40; stages of, 28–29; theory of, 27–29
translator, 30
transportation, transformation and, 27
trauma, 10, 19, 123, 154, 161; acknowledgement of, 165; PTG, 118–119; PTSD, 66; recognition of, 164
tree nuts, 43, 48, 56
tumor, brain, 100
Tylenol, 121
tympanic membranes, 103

ultrasound, 17, 63
urgent care, 79
urinary frequency, 109
urinary urgency, 109–110
urologist, 115
urology, 114
uterus, 112

Van Gogh, Vincent, 104
Veterans Administration, 189
vision: loss of, 12, 185; problems with, 12
vitamin D, 123
vocal cords, 165
voices, of women's health issues, 1–2
vulnerability, 36, 86

Waite Miller, Courtney, 4
walnuts, 48, 56
well-being, sense of, 118
wheat, 43
wheelchair, 87
white privilege, 168
Wilder, Gene, 147
Wilms' tumor, 63, 64
Wit, 209
Womack, Deanna, 5
women: depiction of, 6; health narrative of, 1, 2; treatment of, 79–80; voices of, 1–2
wound care, 180

Xanax, 160

yoga, 153, 154

About the Contributors

Kasey Bruss (BS, University of Wisconsin-Stout) is a graduate of professional communication and emerging media at the University of Wisconsin-Stout, and a mentee of Jennifer Morey Hawkins. Kasey currently is an account coordinator at a digital marketing agency who hopes to eventually use her own health experience and degree to work more closely with pediatric cancer patients.

Krista Calvin (BA, University of Arkansas at Little Rock) is a graduate of communication studies at the University of Arkansas at Little Rock and a mentee of Avinash Thombre.

Jamie Cobb (MA, University of Wyoming) is currently a doctoral student at Wayne State University under the advisement of Dr. Katheryn Maguire. Jamie's scholarly interests are rooted in interpersonal health communication. Specifically, Jamie is interested in the context of chronic illness management within the family and the lived experience of disease management.

Leda Cooks (PhD, Ohio University) is professor in the Department of Communication, University of Massachusetts, Amherst. She teaches dialogue, intercultural communication, and food studies courses from a critical perspective and with a social justice orientation. Her research addresses the ways identity, morality, power, relationships, community, culture, and citizenship intersect in: (1) teaching and learning and (2) producing, preparing, consuming, and communicating about and through food. Her recent work includes essays and research on relational and activist pedagogies, food waste and identities, and a book on food and family over the lifespan.

Ruthann Fox-Hines (PhD, University of North Carolina at Chapel Hill) is retired from the Counseling & Human Development Center at the University of South Carolina in Columbia, South Carolina, and currently in private practice as a licensed counseling psychologist. Her expertise includes individual and group psychotherapy, developing and providing workshops for personal well-being, and interpersonal communication/interaction skills. Dr. Fox-Hines is the author of *Healing the Wound*, a workbook for people dealing with loss.

Jennifer Hall (PhD, Purdue University) is a lecturer and associate director of the online master's program in the Brian Lamb School of Communication. Her training and interests are in health communication, and she has published a book on the role of narrative in understanding high-risk pregnancy.

Laura Hope-Gill (MFA, Warren Wilson College) is assistant professor of writing and director of the Thomas Wolfe Center for Narrative at Lenoir-Rhyne University's Asheville campus. She founded the Certificate in Narrative Healthcare Program in North Carolina, which is grounded in her training in narrative medicine at Columbia University.

Jessica M. W. Kratzer (PhD, University of Missouri) is assistant professor of communication studies at Northern Kentucky University. Her research focuses on women's experiences with childbirth and postpartum issues as well as sexual communication in varying relational contexts.

Robin McIntyre is an advocate for Alzheimer's disease, specifically focused on eliminating the stigma and erasing the fear often associated with Alzheimer's disease. Robin's passion is to continue her mother's legacy in the fight against Alzheimer's through the sharing of her own lived experience. She will never stop sharing her story; not until the first survivor of Alzheimer's disease lives on.

Deleasa Randall-Griffiths (PhD, Southern Illinois University at Carbondale) is associate professor in the Department of Communication Studies and director of the Online Communication Studies Program at Ashland University. Her research interests include health narratives, gender, and women's studies.

Elizabeth Spencer (MA, Pittsburg State University) is a doctoral student in health communication at the University of Kentucky. She is interested in family and interpersonal communication in health contexts.

Wei Sun (PhD, Howard University) is assistant professor in the Department of Communication, Culture and Media Studies, Howard University, Washington, DC. Her scholarly interests are in intercultural communication, new media studies, and health communication.

Avinash Thombe (PhD, University of New Mexico) is professor of communication studies at the University of Arkansas at Little Rock. His primary scholarly interests include health communication, intercultural communication, and understanding the role of self-communication in transformative experiences.

Courtney Waite Miller (PhD, Northwestern University, 2004) is a professor of communication at Elmhurst College. Her recent research focuses on conflict in close relationships and the role this plays in relational, mental, and physical health. She has published in a variety of outlets such as *Communication Yearbook*, *International Journal of Conflict Management*, and *Argumentation and Advocacy*.

Deanna F. Womack (PhD, University of Kansas) is professor of communication and assistant director for organizational & professional communication in the School of Communication and Media at Kennesaw State University. She has published qualitative and quantitative research on conflict management, intercultural communication, health communication, and organizational communication.

ABOUT THE EDITORS

Peter M. Kellett (PhD, Southern Illinois University at Carbondale) is professor of communication studies at the University of North Carolina at Greensboro. His work centers on the various ways that personal narrative methodology can help promote understanding, empowerment, health, and wellness, and a more just and fair world through communication.

Jennifer M. Hawkins (PhD, University of Wisconsin-Milwaukee) is assistant professor of communication studies at St. Cloud State University. Her research focuses on communication occurring with members of underrepresented populations and/or sensitive health topics within interpersonal and intercultural contexts. Believing in the power of narrative to heal, bring forth empathy, and build bridges across differences she utilizes narrative methodology in research and teaching.

www.ingramcontent.com/pod-product-compliance
Lightning Source LLC
Chambersburg PA
CBHW021547020526
44115CB00038B/869